Mastering the
BMAT

Mastering the
BMAT

Christopher Nordstrom
George Rendel
Luke Baxter

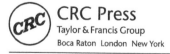

CRC Press
Taylor & Francis Group
Boca Raton London New York

CRC Press is an imprint of the
Taylor & Francis Group, an **informa** business

CRC Press
Taylor & Francis Group
6000 Broken Sound Parkway NW, Suite 300
Boca Raton, FL 33487-2742

© 2017 by Taylor & Francis Group, LLC
CRC Press is an imprint of Taylor & Francis Group, an Informa business

No claim to original U.S. Government works

Printed in Great Britain by Ashford Colour Press Ltd

Version Date: 20160712

International Standard Book Number-13: 978-1-4987-7368-3 (Paperback)

Visit the Taylor & Francis Web site at
http://www.taylorandfrancis.com

and the CRC Press Web site at

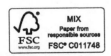

Contents

About the authors

Dr Christopher Nordstrom graduated from University College London with a prize-winning degree in medicine and a first-class honours degree in neuroscience. He undertook medical training in London before starting specialist training in anaesthetics and critical care. Christopher has been involved in medical education for over ten years and has received written praise for his teaching from hospitals and universities, including Imperial College London and University College London. He completed a PgCert in clinical education with distinction and is a Fellow of the Higher Education Academy. His academic achievements include publications in world-renowned journals, published original research and presentations at national and international conferences. He is one of the UK's leading UKCAT and BMAT experts, regularly speaking at national events including the Royal Society of Medicine's Career Day and the Futurewise Careers Day.

George Rendel graduated from the University of Leeds with a prize-winning First Class Degree in English. He went on to work in publishing for Pearson in North America, before continuing his career as a consultant for Accenture in London. George is a co-founder of The Medic Portal, where he is in charge of technology, marketing and content. He is an expert on the verbal reasoning and written components of the BMAT and UKCAT examinations.

Luke Baxter graduated from the University of Cambridge with a first-class degree in Natural Sciences. He has previously worked in France for the international NGO, L'Arche. Currently he is a student on the graduate course in medicine at Cambridge. He also frequently delivers courses on both the UKCAT and BMAT for The Medic Portal.

Introduction

Background

The BioMedical Admissions Test (BMAT) is one of the longest serving aptitude tests used to select prospective medical, dental, veterinary and biomedical sciences students. It is used in the UK and internationally, testing a combination of both aptitude and knowledge.

The BMAT is a two-hour pen and paper test, sat in designated test centres across the world. Most candidates can sit the exam at their school, while school leavers will need to register at their local test centre.

All candidates sit the BMAT on the same date. Usually this is the first Wednesday of November. The results are released three weeks later and remain valid for one year. If a candidate wishes to reapply the following year they will need to resit the BMAT that year.

> **Top Tip:** The BMAT exam takes place *after* you have submitted your university choices via Undergraduate Courses at University and College (UCAS). For medical applicants it is advisable not to apply to more than two BMAT universities to ensure you spread your risk between United Kingdom Clinical Aptitude Test (UKCAT) and BMAT universities.

The BMAT exam is broken into three sections:

- Section 1: Aptitude and Skills
- Section 2: Scientific Knowledge and Applications
- Section 3: Writing Task

Section 1 is the aptitude test. It is designed to test innate problem-solving abilities and does not require any specific factual information. Candidates have to answer 35 multiple choice problem-solving questions, covering mathematical, verbal and spatial reasoning style questions.

Section 2 requires knowledge. It consists of 27 multiple choice science questions covering biology, chemistry, physics and maths. Every year a specific BMAT science syllabus is released, although broadly speaking this covers the sciences to General Certificate of Secondary Education (GCSE) (Key Stage 4) level.

Section 3 is the writing task. Candidates have to write a one A4-sided essay from a choice of four possible question titles. Many students find this task the most daunting – especially as they may have dropped all essay-writing subjects for A levels.

In this book, we will walk you through each of these sections, explaining how they work and what strategies can be adopted to help you score highly. We will be referring to worked examples throughout, and there is a full-length mock exam with model answers at the end of the book.

Courses requiring BMAT

As of Summer 2016, courses requiring the BMAT include:

Medicine:

- Brighton and Sussex Medical School (A100)
- Cambridge University (A100)
- Imperial College London (A100 and A109)
- Keele (non-EU students) (A100 and A104)
- Lancaster University (A100)
- Leeds University (A100)
- Lee Kong Chian School of Medicine (Singapore)
- Oxford University (A100 and A101)
- University College London (A100)

Dentistry:

- Leeds University (A200)

Veterinary Medicine:

- Cambridge University (D100)
- Royal Veterinary College (D100 and D101)

Biomedical Sciences:

- Oxford University (BC98)

There are international variations on the BMAT for specific centres, including BMAT Leiden and BMAT Navarra.

Booking your test

Your test centre will register you for the BMAT; you cannot do this yourself. Most schools and colleges are registered test centres. Current and former pupils should speak to their school or college to register them for the exam. If you are not at school or college you can find registered test centres on the BMAT website to approach. There are test centres located around the world for international applicants.

> **Top Tip:** It is your responsibility to ensure that your test centre registers you for the BMAT exam – make sure you check it has completed this.

Registration opens two months before the exam date (the start of September) and closes one month before the exam. Late entries will be considered for two weeks after the closing date but an additional fee (£32.00) will be levied. The costs of entering the BMAT in 2016 are:

- Standard UK and EU entry: £45
- Non-EU entry: £76

Eligible widening participation candidates can apply to have their standard entry fee reimbursed. This can be claimed back after payment has been made with the appropriate letter of proof. For full criteria, visit the BMAT website.

The test day

It is important to arrive early for your exam. This will ensure you are relaxed and calm, as well as providing a buffer for unexpected delays.

You will need to bring your own writing equipment. For Sections 1 and 2 you will need a **soft pencil** and **eraser**. For Section 3 you will need a pen with **black ink**. You may not bring a calculator or dictionary into the exam hall.

The exam is two hours long. You will be allowed to leave to go to the loo; however, this will use valuable time.

> **Top Tip:** Bring a couple of spare pens and pencils in case they run out.

Extra time and special considerations

Students with certain disabilities may be considered for extra time or the use of a laptop. If you are allowed extra time or laptops for other exams you will need to inform the test centre in advance and bring proof with you.

If you are using a laptop, your Section 3 essay will be limited to 550 words. You must use Arial size 11 font with single spacing. Spell and grammar check software must be disabled throughout.

Non-native English speakers or international applicants do not qualify for extra time, nor may they use a dictionary.

Results and scoring

The BMAT results are released three weeks after the exam. Candidates can log in online to access a breakdown of their results.

Each university uses the BMAT scores in different ways. Some will focus mainly on one or two sections whereas others will consider all three sections. They will each have different cut-offs for deciding who to invite to interview.

In Sections 1 and 2 each question is worth one mark. The raw score is then scaled into a 'BMAT score' ranging from 1 to 9. The scaling is such that average successful candidates will score around 5, strong candidates around 6 and exceptional candidates around 7. Typically only around 3% of candidates score a 7 or above.

Section 3 is marked by two examiners, each of whom grades candidates on the quality of their content (a numerical score from 1 to 5) and the quality of their written English (an alphabetical score of A, C or E). The average of the two examiners is then taken as the final score.

For example, if a candidate scored 5A and 4C from the two examiners, their grade would average as 4.5B. If there is a large discrepancy between the two scores a third examiner will assess the paper.

General technique and strategy

The BMAT exam is tough and requires dedicated revision. Most high-scoring candidates will have spent at least six to eight weeks revising.

All past BMAT papers are available online on the BMAT website. Although the syllabus has changed, the 2003 to 2008 papers are still useful.

The Medic Portal website (www.themedicportal.com) hosts a fully interactive BMAT question bank, in which you can answer hundreds of questions from each section and instantly get feedback and worked solutions. It even includes BMAT essay tasks with model notes and responses.

Top Tip: Save the last three years' worth of papers to practise to time closer to your exam date.

Each section will require independent revision, testing different skills. For Section 1 you will need to practise solving mathematical problems without the comfort of a calculator. For those applying to medicine and dentistry you will find that sitting the UKCAT will help with some of the verbal and mathematical aspects.

Each year an official BMAT science guide is published. There is an online e-book along with syllabus stipulating all areas you must cover. Some topics in the BMAT syllabus are not present on all GCSE syllabuses, so make sure you go through the BMAT syllabus to ensure you have revised all potential topics.

Top Tip: There is no negative marking in the BMAT. Sections 1 and 2 are both multiple choice. If you find yourself running out of time make educated guesses to ensure you've answered all questions.

Section 3 can be daunting – especially if you are no longer studying essay-based subjects. It is important to print out sample answer sheets from the BMAT website and use these when practising questions. This lets you familiarise yourself with the format you will encounter on the day and allows you to practise with the space constraints.

Timing is tight but with practice most students find they will finish each section. It is important that if you are stuck on a question to move on – remember each question is only worth one mark.

General Top Tips:

- Ensure you cover the theoretical knowledge required for the exam.
- Use the BMAT syllabus to structure your revision.
- Never leave a question blank – there is no negative marking.
- Structure a revision plan over six to eight weeks for optimal results.
- Make sure you do all the past papers available online.
- Practise sections to time – including the essay.

Problem solving, spatial reasoning and verbal reasoning

Overview

The first section of the BMAT exam is designed to test aptitude. It does not require any specific knowledge, but instead is designed to assess your problem-solving abilities. Broadly speaking, questions cover logic and mathematical skills, and verbal and spatial reasoning abilities. You are, however, expected to have a solid grasp of basic mathematical principles up to GCSE level.

Format of the section

Section 1 contains 35 multiple choice questions to be answered in 60 minutes. This equates to approximately 103 seconds per question. In reality, some questions will take much longer whereas others are quite quick.

You must answer the questions on the computer-read answer sheet provided using a pencil. If you mark more than one answer option per question, you will not score any points.

Top Tip: If changing your answers, make sure you rub them out completely to prevent the computer reading two answers and therefore scoring you zero points.

Every question is worth one mark and there is no negative marking. It is therefore vital that you do not leave any questions unanswered. Competition is tight and approximately 25% of candidates will score within three marks of each other. Therefore, one mark could be the difference between success and failure.

Problem solving and verbal reasoning typically each make up approximately a third of Section 1, with the remainder of questions covering spatial reasoning and data analysis (which could include verbal, statistical and graphical information).

Question format

The questions will take one of two formats:

- Single answer
- Combination answer

Single answer questions consist of a question stem, followed by three or more answer options. Combination answer questions contain a stem, three possible answer statements and then three or more answer options involving different combinations of the answer statements.

There will also be a few longer 'question sets'. These questions contain a large amount of information, often a combination of text and tables or graphs followed by four questions. These can be purely verbal, logical or mathematical, but often contain a mixture of question types.

Top Tip: The longer question types don't usually require you to read all the information. The questions will point you towards the relevant part of the information.

Verbal reasoning

Verbal reasoning questions make up approximately a third of Section 1 questions. They are predominantly designed to test your understanding of arguments. It helps to have studied critical thinking when approaching these questions.

The majority of questions are single or combination answer questions, although there will usually be a few verbal reasoning questions linked to a longer question set format.

Top Tip: The BMAT Section 1 verbal questions are similar to the UKCAT 'new format' comprehension style questions.

The basic format of the verbal reasoning single answer questions is:

1. 100 to 150-word argument (the passage)

2. A question

3. Four or five answer options

The combination answer questions are similar, and consist of:

1. 100 to 150-word argument (the passage)

2. A question

3. Three statements

4. Three to seven answer options made from combinations of the three statements

Understanding arguments

Before attempting to answer verbal reasoning questions it's important to understand the basic principles of an argument. In its simplest form, an argument is a set of reasons given in support of an idea or theory. In addition, you must be familiar with the definition of:

- Premises
- Conclusions
- Assumptions
- Flaws

A premise is a previous statement or proposition from which another is inferred or follows as a conclusion. A conclusion is a proposition that is reached from given premise(s). In other words, a premise can be thought of as the 'evidence' or 'supporting statement' used to justify an overall conclusion.

Below is an example of an argument:

> Regular exercise reduces the rate of atherosclerosis, which in turn reduces your chance of suffering a heart attack. In addition, exercise releases endorphins which have a positive effect on mood and psychological well-being. People who exercise regularly have longer life expectancies than those with sedentary lifestyles. Therefore, exercise is beneficial to your health.

From the above example we can see that there are three premises leading to an overall conclusion:

- Exercise reduces rates of atherosclerosis and therefore heart attacks.
- Exercise improves mood through the release of endorphins. ⎫
- Regular exercise is linked to longer life expectancy.   ⎬ Premises
- Exercise is beneficial to health.   } Conclusion

When explaining arguments (and related questions) we will refer to the famous ancient Greek palace – the Parthenon. Visualising arguments as the Parthenon will allow you to understand how they can be attacked or strengthened.

Consider a basic argument as the Parthenon:

Just as the roof of the Parthenon is supported by the pillars, the conclusion of an argument is supported by the premises.

In Section 1 verbal reasoning there are five question formats you will encounter where you will need to identify:

- Conclusions
- Assumptions
- Flaws
- Strengthening arguments
- Weakening arguments

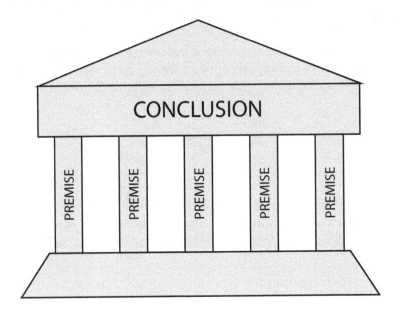

Conclusions

A conclusion is the proposition that is reached from given premise(s). It is important to differentiate between **a** conclusion and **the** conclusion.

A conclusion is, simply speaking, something that **logically follows** on from the premises. Logically follows means you cannot help but reach a particular conclusion without making any assumptions. In other words, you have not had to make any assumptions or use any outside knowledge.

Consider the following statement:

In the kitchen there are two apples in the fridge, two in the fruit bowl and none anywhere else.

It therefore logically follows that there **must** be four apples in the kitchen. Although not explicitly stated, you know this for a fact.

A conclusion is therefore simply something that logically follows from the passage. It is similar to 'true' in UKCAT verbal reasoning. This differs from questions asking you to identify **the** conclusion. *The* conclusion (sometimes referred to as **the main conclusion**) means the 'point' of the argument as a whole.

> **Top Tip:** Remember passages can have more than one conclusion, as technically many statements can logically follow from the premises. **The**, or **the main**, conclusion is the **'point'** of the whole argument. Be careful to assess all answer options before committing to an answer.

Question 1

One of the biggest issues facing societies in advanced economies around the world is disconnect between urban and rural areas. Traditionally, as a country's economy develops, the social separation between urban and rural populations widens. Attitudes towards hunting are an excellent example of an ideological schism that can occur in such cases. In rural societies, growing food, slaughtering animals and hunting for sport are often everyday occurrences. And someone who slaughters a pig for their family to eat would see little wrong with spending their leisure time killing animals. Yet, in urban environments, where societies are typically further removed from any of the processes used to produce the food they consume, many are horrified at the idea of hunting for sport.

What conclusion can be drawn from the above passage?

A. Urban societies are unaware of how their food is produced.

B. Rural populations are less affected by changes in economic development.

C. Differences in opinion can be shaped by an individual's experience.

D. Hunting for sport is not seen as acceptable by urban populations.

E. Economic development often results in an improvement in animal rights.

Question 1: answer and explanation

The passage states that 'someone who slaughters a pig for their family to eat would see little wrong with then spending their leisure time killing animals'. It goes on to say that 'in urban environments, where societies are typically further removed from any of the processes used to produce the food they consume, many are horrified at the idea of hunting for sport'. This represents a difference of opinion that is shaped by individual experience. The correct answer is therefore C.

A is incorrect because the passage does not say that urban populations are unaware of how their food is produced – just that they are more removed from the processes.

B is incorrect because the passage does not present any evidence that rural populations are less affected by changes in economic development.

D is incorrect because the passage does not state that urban populations as a whole, and in their entirety, view hunting for sport as 'unacceptable'.

E is incorrect because the passage does not discuss the issue of animal rights.

Top Tip: Make sure you don't confuse a premise with a conclusion. Representing the argument as the Parthenon will help you avoid this pitfall.

Value judgements

Some verbal reasoning questions introduce value judgements. This is where you need to decide which option is 'more correct' than the other options. It therefore means that several options could be theoretically correct, but you need to make an assessment of rightness or wrongness to gauge which option is the best fit.

Value judgement questions are signalled by words such as 'best' or 'most' in the question. For example:

Which of the following is the **best** conclusion of the above passage?

Reading this question should immediately alert you to the fact that more than one answer option might technically represent a valid conclusion that logically follows from the passage. You need to make a value judgement as to which option is the most suitable. Usually this is the option with the highest 'impact factor'. In other words, the option that is the main conclusion.

Assumptions

An assumption is a thing that is accepted as true or certain to happen, but without proof. Assumptions can therefore be considered as unstated premises:

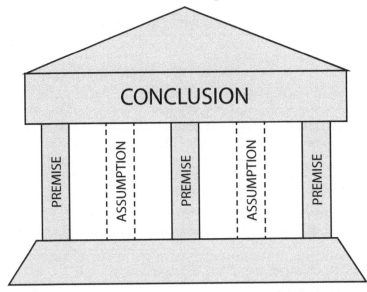

The Parthenon model shows us that assumptions are 'see-through pillars'. They must be present in order for the argument to hold true; however, they are not explicitly stated within the passage.

Assumption questions usually ask you to identify which of the answer options is/are assumptions in the argument. It can be useful to use the following algorithm when assessing each answer option in turn to decide whether a statement is an assumption or not:

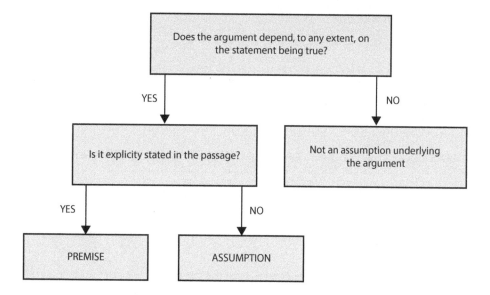

Question 2

In some countries, it is illegal not to participate in a general election. The decision not to vote can even lead to the individual in question receiving a fine. This is often seen as a good thing, as it leads to more people being interested in politics. Naturally, if someone has to vote no matter what, they will take an added interest in the political climate. Compulsory voting also reduces the potential of governments to ignore minority groups, due to the fact that a certain demographic is unlikely to hold them to account at the ballot box.

Which of the following is an assumption in the above argument?

A. Some countries have different voting laws than others.

B. Governments ignore minority groups if not held to account.

C. There is a correlation between voting and political interest.

D. Fewer people will vote if they are not legally compelled to do so.

E. Penalising those who do not vote is a good thing.

Question 2: answer and explanation

The passage claims that 'if someone has to vote no matter what, they will take an added interest in the political climate'. This statement shows that the author is linking voting to political interest. Since this link is not demonstrated, it is an assumption. It is also a questionable one, since it does not account for people who may vote purely to avoid financial penalties. The correct answer is therefore C.

A is incorrect because voting laws are a matter of fact and therefore not based on assumption.

B is incorrect because the passage only says that the laws reduce the 'potential' of this happening.

D is incorrect because this is not an assumption underlying the argument about voter interest and government actions.

E is incorrect because the passage only says that it is often seen that way; it does not assume it to be true.

Argument flaws

An argument flaw is an imperfection, often concealed, that impairs the soundness of an argument. It is important to remember that a flaw does not necessarily render the conclusion incorrect – it simply introduces an imperfection that increases the likelihood it may be wrong.

Consider the Parthenon:

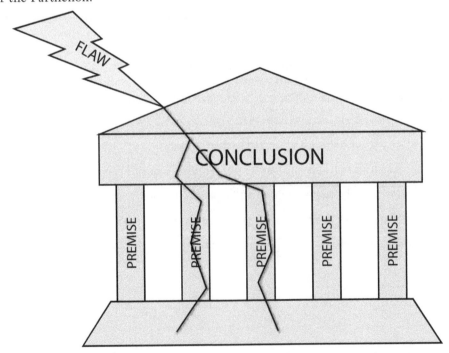

If the Parthenon were to be struck by lightning, cracks may develop in the structure. These cracks won't necessarily cause the building to collapse, but will certainly affect the soundness of the structure. Similarly, if a flaw were to be introduced into an argument the conclusion may still hold true, although the soundness would certainly be impaired.

There are well over 100 types of flaw (also known as fallacies) described in critical thinking. But for the BMAT the main types encountered are:

- Flaw of causation
- Conflation
- Straw man fallacy
- Ad hominem
- Bifurcation fallacy
- Generalisations
- Circular reasoning

Flaw of causation

This usually means confusing correlation with causation. It assumes that because two events happen in close proximity, there must be a causal link between them. Consider the following example:

> More people who take paracetamol develop brain tumours. Therefore, we can conclude that paracetamol causes brain tumours.

It may very well be the case that more people taking paracetamol develop brain tumours. But this conclusion assumes that there is a direct link between the two, despite there being no concrete evidence for this.

It fails to take into account the fact that there might be other factors involved. Maybe those with brain tumours develop frequent headaches, therefore take more paracetamol? Or perhaps people with brain tumours consume more paracetamol *as a result* of the tumour, rather than as a precursor to it developing.

Top Tip: Correlation does not necessarily mean causation!

Conflation

Conflation relates to flawed analogies. These is sometimes colloquially known as 'comparing apples and oranges'. This is when an argument compares two or more concepts, treating them as the same thing when in reality they are not. Consider the argument below:

Last year 1000 UK citizens died in car crashes while only 25 died in plane crashes. Therefore, planes are four times as safe as cars.

This argument attempts to compare the safety of cars and planes. However, the comparison is flawed because we do not know how many journeys were made by each mode of transport. If only 25 flights were taken, the mortality rate was in fact 100%! In other words, we might be comparing apples and oranges.

Straw man fallacy

The straw man fallacy is when the arguer misrepresents an argument and cites premises and conclusions that were not in fact made by the person he is arguing against. The argument below highlights the straw man fallacy:

Individual 1: We should limit immigration to help boost the job prospects of our unemployed youth.

Individual 2: Individual 1 thinks that we should ban immigration, not do anything to help those disadvantaged in other countries and instead let them continue to live in poverty.

In this case, Individual 2 has misrepresented the argument put forward by Individual 1. Did Individual 1 say we should ban immigration? Did they say we should not do anything to help others living in poverty in other countries? By misrepresenting the argument, Individual 2 has made it easier to attack the argument.

Ad hominem

This is when someone seeks to undermine an argument by attacking the character of the individual delivering it. For example:

Paul believes that to make the country safer all guns should be banned. This is ironic, as Paul used to go hunting with his dad as a child. How can we take Paul's argument seriously?

Paul may have a well-thought-out and logical argument, but the arguer has attacked Paul's personal circumstances, rather than the soundness of the argument.

Bifurcation fallacy

The bifurcation fallacy is also known as 'restricting the options' or 'false dilemma'. It arises when the argument forces an individual to choose between a narrow range of options, when in reality there is at least one other viable option. An example of this is as follows:

The universe must either have arisen as the result of the Big Bang, an infinitely small and dense point which exploded outwards, or have been formed by a divine Creator, as it could not have arisen from nothing. As a Creator would also have needed to arise from something, the Big Bang is the most plausible explanation.

This argument does not take into account any other theories or options, but instead assumes that only one of the two listed options must be true. There could be many other theories which offer viable explanations.

Generalisations

Generalisations occur when arguments extrapolate specific points into general theories. This leads to flaws. Although the specific point may be representative of all cases, it is likely that it is not. As a result, incorrect conclusions may be drawn. For example:

When visiting Sweden on holiday, the people who caught my eye all had blond hair. Therefore, all Swedish people have blond hair.

While it may be true that relatively speaking there are more blond-haired individuals in Sweden, it is incorrect to generalise it into 'all'.

Circular reasoning

Circular reasoning occurs when an argument assumes that what you are trying to prove is true, or when the conclusion is used as a premise. These arguments are flawed. It's just like someone telling you: *I'm right because I'm right!*

Question 3

Medical professionals frequently lament a lack of availability when it comes to donor organs. One idea for addressing this is that eligibility to receive organ transplants be limited only to those who themselves are registered as organ donors. This would offer a practical solution to the lack of organ donors, as people would probably not want to be refused the chance for potentially life-saving surgery. And it stands to reason that organ donors are more deserving of organs, as they are prepared to offer up their own. So, this new policy, if introduced, would create a virtuous cycle, whereby there would be more organ donors, and organ donors themselves would always get an organ if needed.

Which of the following could be a flaw in the above argument?

A. It uses the term 'virtuous cycle' without defining it.

B. It confuses donor numbers with organ availability.

C. It doesn't account for large administration costs associated with adding people to the donor register.

D. There is no legal way of defining if someone is deserving of an organ.

E. It is wrong to punish someone so severely for one mistake.

Question 3: answer and explanation

The passage concludes that making organs available only to donors would mean donors would always get an organ. However, this is not mathematically true, since a donor does not necessarily mean an available organ. And, even if it did, if the number of donors in need outweighed the number of donors in a position to provide, the 'virtuous cycle' would not work. The correct answer is therefore B.

A is incorrect because this term does not need to be defined for the argument to be valid – only used correctly.

C is incorrect because the argument is not concerned with costs.

D is incorrect because it is not relevant to the argument presented.

E is incorrect because the argument does not consider the moral implications of the policy.

Structural flaws

The above examples have all looked at content flaws. But BMAT Section 1 also uses arguments with structural flaws (sometimes known as 'reasoning errors'). For example:

All humans are mammals. Therefore, all mammals are humans.

Sometimes, if you want to understand the structure of an argument, it helps to translate it into letters. In this case, that would give us:

All A is B. Therefore, all B is A.

This is obviously an incorrect conclusion to draw from the information provided.

Top Tip: Putting the argument structure into letters allows you to spot structural flaws more easily.

Question 4

Daniel Day-Lewis is the only actor in history to have won three Oscars for Best Actor. He took the prestigious Academy Award in 1989, 2007 and 2012 for *My Left Foot*, *There Will be Blood* and *Lincoln* respectively. Many people think this makes him the best actor in the world. Day-Lewis is a well-known exponent of the 'method' school of acting, whose members also include Marlon Brando and Robert De Niro, who at various times have also been considered the best actors in the world. To be considered the best actor in the world, it is therefore necessary to be a 'method' actor.

Which of the following makes the same reasoning error as the above argument?

A. Most pieces of music are only as good as the musician who performs them.

B. Fernando is a Spanish singer, so to be a singer you must be Spanish.

C. All cats are mammals, therefore all mammals are cats.

D. Most Ferraris are red, so the majority of red cars are Ferraris.

Question 4: answer and explanation

The format of the argument is: A is B. A is C. Therefore, to be B you must be C. The correct answer is B.

A has the format: A depends on B.

C has the format: All A is B. Therefore all B is C.

D has the format: Most A is B. Therefore most B is A.

> **Top Tip:** When trying to identify the flaw in an argument think like a detective and work backwards from the conclusion to the premises. By finding the illogical 'jump' in logic you have identified the flaw in the argument.

Strengthening and weakening the argument

Frequently, questions will ask you to select which statement will either strengthen or weaken the argument in the passage. These questions are easier to approach if you think about the Parthenon model.

To strengthen an argument, you can either add another premise or strengthen an existing premise. Below is an example of a short argument to show how you can strengthen a premise:

Passage: Mr Daniels must be a good physics teacher as last year 75% of his students scored an A★ in GCSE physics.

Statement: After remarking, it turned out that in fact 82% of Mr Daniels' students achieved an A★ grade.

We can see that the statement will strengthen the argument, as it solidifies an existing premise (in this case the high number of A★ grades achieved).

Thinking of the Parthenon model, this would mean adding another pillar or increasing the size of an existing pillar – both have the result of strengthening the foundation of the building.

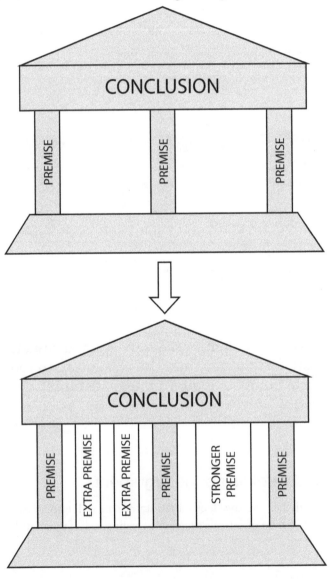

Weakening the argument relies on the same principles as strengthening the argument – but in reverse. You can weaken an argument by either removing a premise or by introducing a flaw. Remember, a flaw doesn't necessarily render the conclusion incorrect, but it does decrease the likelihood of the conclusion being right.

In terms of the Parthenon model you can weaken the argument by removing a pillar or by introducing a 'crack'. Both of these weaken the foundations of the structure.

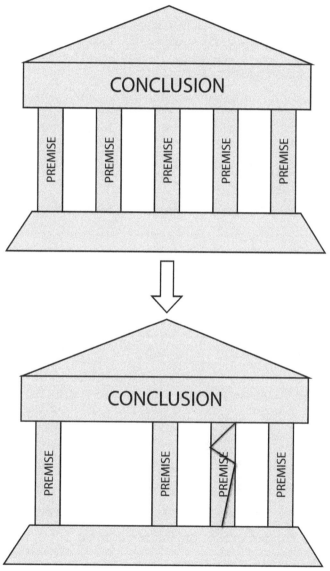

Top Tip: By learning the different types of flaw that can be introduced into arguments you will understand how to approach both 'flaw' and 'weakening' style questions.

Question 5

Many people are quick to call potential ministers of political parties `career politicians'. This term is used as a way of negativity labelling a candidate, based upon the idea that politics is their chosen career and that being elected is a mere stepping stone in their career path, rather than a genuine opportunity to represent their constituency. But this label is an archaic one. We no longer live in a world where politicians are made up of generous individuals who are willing to give up their time to represent the needs of others. Politics is a serious business and we need the best people for the job, regardless of their background. Therefore, those who seek out a career as a politician should be applauded, not chastised due to criticisms founded on dubious assumptions.

Which of the following, if true, would most weaken the argument presented?

A. The best politicians often benefit from skills they acquired from a range of professions and environments.

B. People who have had successful careers outside of politics often do not face financial pressures when campaigning to become a politician.

C. Every political candidate must pass a background check before they can be considered for election.

D. It is rare to be a good politician and be unpopular.

E. The idea of following a career solely in politics is relatively recent.

Question 5: answer and explanation

The passage implies that `career politicians' should be applauded based on the premise that `politics is a serious business and we need the best people for the job, regardless of their background'. If 'A' were true, it would suggest that `career politicians' may not be as suited to the job as other candidates, thereby justifying many of the concerns that this argument seeks to dismiss. The correct answer is therefore A.

B is incorrect because the issue of financial independence is not relevant to the argument.

C is incorrect because the issue of a background check is not relevant to the argument.

D is incorrect because the argument does not say that all career politicians are unpopular.

E is incorrect because it agrees with the argument presented.

Types of evidence

There are five different types of evidence you need to understand for the BMAT exam:

1. Conclusive evidence: This is strong factual evidence, often derived from research and experiments, which cannot be contradicted by the other types of evidence.

2. Statistical evidence: This is evidence based on numbers and samples. It can be very strong (if you have a large, representative sample) but can be exploited to falsely demonstrate an effect by using a small, non-representative sample.

3. Anecdotal evidence: This is evidence based on personal accounts and observations, not research or scientific study. Generally speaking it is a weak form of evidence.

4. Hearsay: This is unofficial, unverified information gained from someone else and not part of one's direct knowledge. Hearsay is a weak form of evidence as it cannot be corroborated.

5. Irrelevant evidence: This is evidence that is cited in support of an idea or theory but which has no actual relevance to the argument. It is therefore a very weak form of evidence.

You may be asked to identify what type of evidence has been used in a particular argument.

Glossary of argument terminology

- Argument: A persuasive piece of text or speech consisting of premises leading to a conclusion.
- Assumption: Something that is accepted as true or certain to happen, but without proof.
- Conclusion: A proposition that is reached from given premise(s).
- Correlation: Two or more events regularly occur in close proximity. Correlation does not necessarily imply causation.
- Evidence: Factual material used in support of a claim.
- Flaw: An argument flaw is an imperfection, often concealed, that impairs the soundness of an argument.
- Inference: Moving from premise(s) to a conclusion.
- Logically follows: You cannot help but reach a particular conclusion without making any assumptions.
- Premise: A statement or proposition from which another is inferred or follows as a conclusion.
- Value judgement: Assessing the rightness or wrongness of something.

Logical and mathematical reasoning

The problem-solving questions in Section 1 can be very tricky. There are some recurring themes and styles of questions which repeat, but each year there will usually be one or two completely new question varieties.

These questions are designed to assess your ability to apply logic and reasoning to solve problems. It is about figuring out the underlying principles in the question – something which can be hard to do in the time allowed.

In the remainder of this chapter, we will run through some of the common themes and underlying principles involved in these questions, and will highlight how they work in practice with sample questions.

> **Top Tip:** Be careful of time. It is easy to spend too long trying to solve one problem. This has a domino effect that may well see you run out of time on the remaining questions.

Time and date questions

Time and date questions are common and, if understood, can be very quick to answer. Therefore, they can offer a steady source of marks.

Question 6

Four of my friends are called Jasmine, Fiona, Liam and Minaj. Their birthdays are on the 77th, 177th, 200th and 312th day of the year respectively.

Which two of my friends will have their birthday on the same day of the week as each other?

A. Jasmine and Fiona

B. Jasmine and Liam

C. Jasmine and Minaj

D. Fiona and Liam

E. Fiona and Minaj

F. Liam and Minaj

Question 6: answer and explanation

Time and date questions are relatively straightforward. In this case, in order to have their birthdays on the same day of the week, the difference in number of days between two of the friends' birthdays must be divisible by seven. This is because there are seven days in a week. If the difference is not divisible by seven, the birthdays cannot be on the same day.

Liam and Minaj have their birthdays on the 200th and 312th day respectively. The difference is 112, which is divisible by 7 (112 / 7 = 16). They will therefore have their birthdays on the same day of the week, 16 weeks apart.

Top Tip: If the question is looking for months of the year, find a difference divisible by 12.

Partial table questions

Partial table questions provide you with a table of information which is only partially completed. The introductory text will usually establish a set of 'rules' for how the table operates and how it should be filled in. You will need to complete the table in order to answer the question.

Top Tip: Pay close attention to the rules provided. There is sufficient information provided to answer the questions, although there may not be enough to complete the whole table.

Question 7

Paul, Matt, Susan and Orpa are attending a training day with four different sessions. A trainee cannot attend all four sessions and each session must have at least two trainees attending. Paul and Susan each attend only one session.

The session planner starts the following table:

	Morning	Afternoon	Evening	Night
Paul		✓		
Matt			✗	
Susan				
Orpa			✓	

Which sessions does Matt attend?

A. Morning and Afternoon

B. Morning, Afternoon and Night

C. Morning and Night

D. Afternoon only

E. Afternoon and Night

F. Night only

Question 7: answer and explanation

All the rules needed to complete the table are provided. Paul only attends one session so he does not attend the morning, evening or night sessions. Each session must have at least two trainees so Susan must attend the evening session. Susan does not attend the morning, afternoon or night sessions (as she only attends one session). Consequently Matt and Orpa both attend the morning and night sessions as each session requires two attendees. A trainee cannot attend all four sessions; hence Orpa does not attend the afternoon session, meaning that Matt must attend the afternoon session.

Matt therefore attends the morning, afternoon and night sessions.

	Morning	Afternoon	Evening	Night
Paul	✗	✓	✗	✗
Matt	✓	✓	✗	✓
Susan	✗	✗	✓	✗
Orpa	✓	✗	✓	✓

Top Tip: You can use the table in your question booklet to tick and cross as you go along, saving time when compared to drawing out the table.

PIN number questions

PIN numbers lend themselves to generating logical reasoning questions using numbers. There are usually two parts to these questions:

1. Use logical reasoning to deduce the correct PIN number.

2. Solve one or more of the PIN numbers then apply basic calculations on the numbers.

Question 8

The four digits of the PIN number of my debit card are all different and, when written out as words, in alphabetical order. When the digits are written as words, I find that the first letter is different for each digit. The sum of any two digits will always be less than 15. The third digit of my PIN is 7.

What is the total number of letters required to spell the first three digits of my PIN number?

A. 10

B. 11

C. 12

D. 13

E. 14

F. 15

Question 8: answer and explanation

PIN number questions rely on using only 10 numbers:

1. Zero

2. One

3. Two

4. Three

5. Four

6. Five

7. Six

8. Seven

9. Eight

10. Nine

When written out as words it is easy to spot characteristics that will allow you to eliminate them as options:

- The number of letters
- The first letter

The third digit is 7 and the sum of any two numbers must be less than 15 so my PIN does not include 8 or 9 (otherwise the sum would be greater than 15). The first letter of each digit begins with a different letter when written as a word so my PIN does not include 6 (as both 6 and 7 begin with S). For this reason, only one of 4 and 5 can be included (both begin with the letter F). This means that the 1 must be included (as this is the only number left since 0, 2 or 3 would all be after 7 since the PIN is in alphabetical order).

Since the digits are in alphabetical order, the first letter of each digit in order will either be FOST or FOSZ. Both 4 and 5 have the same number of letters (four). Hence the total number of letters for the first three digits is 12.

In this case, you do not need to know if the PIN starts with a 4 or 5 – and it is impossible to tell based on the information.

Number sequence questions

It is common to encounter number sequence questions. These usually require you to break down a sequence using a set of 'rules' provided in the question. The second step will require logical reasoning to decipher the answer, often combining the theory from 'time and date' questions.

Question 9

A spy ring uses a code whereby each letter is given a numerical value (A = 1, B = 2, C = 3, etc.) and a word is ended by giving the cumulative total of the letters in that word. The cumulative total 'resets' to zero at the beginning of a new word.

For example, 'COW' would be '3152341' because the letters of the word equal 3, 15 and 23 respectively giving cumulative totals of 41 (3 + 15 + 23).

The ring leaders receive a string of numbers from one of their agents, which translates into a single word (in English). However, the string of numbers is repeated, so the leaders are unsure where the number broadcast begins and ends.

Here is a transcript of the repeated section: 1255480252018

What are the first and last letters of the word?

A. U and S

B. M and E

C. B and D

D. G and M

E. F and S

Question 9: answer and explanation

This question could probably be answered through trial and error until you identify letters that 'work', but this may take up precious time. A quick way to do it is to spot that zero can never appear as the first digit in a number (see the example, 'C' is represented as '3'). Whenever a zero appears it must either represent the letters J or T (numerical values 10 and 20 respectively), or it must be a digit in the cumulative total. We have two zeros – one preceded by an eight, the other preceded by a two.

There are 13 digits in the string of numbers above – note that the highest value possible in a string of 13 digits is 130, the total of five 'Z's – 2626262626130 (the code for 'ZZZZZ'). Therefore, 80 *must* be the cumulative total in the string of digits above because it contains a zero *and* it is the highest digit-combination that is lower than 130.

This must mean that the zero preceded by a two is 20 or 'T'. From here it is easy to work out the rest of the string:

- 25201812554 arranged as numbers added together must equal 80.
- 25T1812554 – note that 25, 'Y', rarely precedes T so more likely to be B, E.
- B, E, T, 1812554 – note that 55 and 54 cannot be letters, so final two digits must be E and D.
- B, E, T, 18125 E, D; 80 – (2 + 5 + 20 + 5 + 4) = 44.
- 18125 could be: AHABE or AHAY or RLE or RAY or RABE.

Only RAY fits – so the word is 'BETRAYED', although obviously you should stop when you know the first and final letters! The correct answer is therefore C.

Travel

Logical reasoning questions involving travelling and distances are common. It is essential that you are familiar with:

$$speed = \frac{distance}{time}$$

You may also be expected to interpret graphs using the gradient and area under the graph.

Top Tip: In a **velocity-time** graph the area under the graph is equal to the distance travelled.

Question 10

There are 26 stations, labelled from A to Z. A train moving at 100 mph passes through Station A, heading towards Station Z. A car moving at 60 mph passes Station F, also heading towards Station Z.

If Stations A to Z are spaced apart in a straight line, with a constant distance of 10 miles between each station, when will the train overtake the car?

A. At Station L

B. Between Station L and M

C. Between Station M and N

D. At Station N

Question 10: answer and explanation

The car has a 50-mile head start on the train. The train is moving 100 – 60 = 40 mph faster than the car. Therefore, it will close the 50 mile gap within 50/40 = 1.25 hours.

In this time, the car will have advanced 60 x 1.25 = 75 miles. So, if it started at Station F, it will be halfway between stations M and N when the train catches it.

(To check, you can see where the train will be after 1.25 hours; it has moved 125 miles which, if you divide by 10, gets you 12.5 stations away from A, which is halfway between M and N.)

Top Tip: It is important to remember that the focus of these questions is on problem solving, rather than mathematical ability. Pure maths skills will be tested in Section 2. In Section 1, the focus is on thinking logically around the problem to generate the answer.

Question 11

As part of a celebration, two antique steam trains are heading along straight tracks towards a station where they arrive simultaneously. One train comes from the north while one comes from the south travelling at 25 and 45 mph respectively. The initial distance between the trains is 70 miles.

A helicopter, flying at 65 mph is filming the events. The helicopter sets off from the southern station at the same time as the train, following the railway tracks towards the other train. When it reaches the northern train it turns around and heads back to the southern train. It then turns around again heading back to the northern train and continues doing this until the trains meet.

How far will the helicopter have flown by the time the trains meet?

A. 65 miles

B. 70 miles

C. 90 miles

D. 110 miles

E. 135 miles

F. Can't tell

Question 11: answer and explanation

On the surface this question looks difficult. The key thing to remember is that when a question looks disproportionately convoluted there is usually a simpler way of solving it through logic.

You know that the two trains are 70 miles apart and will be heading towards each other at 25 + 45 = 70 mph. Using time = distance / speed we can calculate that the trains will meet in 1 hour.

The helicopter which is filming the events is travelling at 65 mph. So, the key question is simply: how far will a helicopter fly when travelling at 65 mph for 1 hour? Suddenly the problem has become easy to answer! The answer is therefore A – 65 miles.

Top Tip: Although questions may look mathematical, they may simply be testing some basic logical reasoning and problem-solving skills.

Graphs and data analysis

There will usually be three to five questions based around interpreting graphs and data. We will cover more on this in later chapters (Section 2 – Maths). Often data interpretation and graphical questions will form part of longer question sets, where there will be four follow-on questions from one set of data.

You will need to be comfortable interpreting:

- Line graphs
- Bar charts
- Pie charts
- Histograms
- Box plots
- Venn diagrams
- Scatter diagrams
- Cumulative frequency graphs

All of the above are covered in detail in subsequent chapters (Section 2 – Maths).

Question 12

The following scatter graph shows data for several different countries. The x-axis shows the average alcohol intake, in units, per week per adult member of the population. The y-axis displays the incidence of liver disease per 100 000 of the population. The scale starts at zero on both axes.

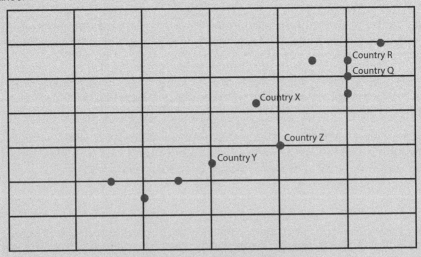

Below are five statements related to the scatter graph above:

1. Alcohol intake may cause liver disease.

2. If Country Y has an incidence of liver disease of 1230 per hundred thousand, Country Z has an incidence of 1640 per hundred thousand.

3. Out of all the countries displayed, Country X has the median incidence of liver disease per hundred thousand of adult population.

4. Liver disease might not come as a result of increased alcohol intake.

5. Country Q has the modal incidence of liver disease per hundred thousand of population.

Which of the following statements is/are consistent with what is displayed on the scatter graph?

A. 1 only

B. 1 and 2

C. 2 and 3

D. 3 and 5

E. 1, 2 and 3

F. 1, 3 and 4

G. 2, 3 and 5

H. 3, 4 and 5

I. 1, 2, 4 and 5

J. All of the above

Question 12: answer and explanation

This is an example of a question that tests your ability to interpret scatter diagrams. It is also a combination answer style question.

Assessing each answer option in turn:

1. This is consistent with what is presented on the graph. The scatter of the points suggests that there is some association between liver disease and alcohol intake, and this might be the relationship at work.

2. Incidence of liver disease is expressed on the y-axis, so if Country Y has an incidence of 1230 per hundred thousand, Country Z has an incidence of (1230/5) x 6 = 1476 per hundred thousand, so this statement is incorrect.

3. Country X is the sixth out of 11 data points on the graph ascending the y-axis, so it does show the median incidence of liver disease per hundred thousand out of the countries displayed.

4. This is true: there might be a third variable that links alcohol intake and liver disease which could explain the association seen on the graph.

5. Country Q has the modal incidence of alcohol intake, not liver disease incidence (which is what Country R displays) – so this statement is incorrect.

The correct answer is therefore F – 1, 3 and 4.

Working without a calculator

One of the challenges of the BMAT exam is working without a calculator. In addition to basic arithmetic, you need to be comfortable working with orders of magnitude:

Prefix	Factor	Symbol	Decimal Equivalent
Tera	10^{12}	T	1,000,000,000,000
Giga	10^{9}	G	1,000,000,000
Mega	10^{6}	M	1,000,000
Kilo	10^{3}	K	1000
Hecto	10^{2}	h	100
Deca	10^{1}	da	10
	10^{0}		1
Deci	10^{-1}	d	0.1
Centi	10^{-2}	c	0.01
Milli	10^{-3}	m	0.001
Micro	10^{-6}	μ	0.000 001
Nano	10^{-9}	n	0.000 000 001

Although unlikely to appear as a standalone question, you may need to quickly add a large quantity of numbers together, or calculate an average as part of a question. Consider the following scenario:

The scores of 10 students in a chemistry test are listed below:

54, 76, 64, 56, 72, 90, 38, 50, 55, 64

What was their total combined score?

    A. 616

    B. 619

    C. 622

    D. 624

    E. 630

Although you could spend valuable time adding the numbers together, there are two tricks you can use to quickly eliminate answer options:

1. **Add the last digit of each number in the question.** By adding the last digit of each value, you know what number the final total ends in. You can then select the correct answer by process of elimination.

2. **Odds and evens.** In the above number sequence there is only one odd number – so the answer must be odd! There is only one odd answer option, B, so this must be correct.

> **Top Tip:** If you have an odd number of odd numbers, your answer must be odd!

Spatial reasoning

The spatial reasoning questions in BMAT can be tricky and time consuming. It's important to keep an eye on your timings, as it's easy to get carried away trying to solve just one question.

The spatial reasoning questions can be broadly split into three categories:

- Hidden objects and visualisation
- Construction and deconstruction
- Navigation

Some questions will combine elements of two – or even three – of the above categories.

Hidden objects and visualisation

As a doctor you will need to be able to mentally visualise what structures should look like when performing procedures, and increasingly be able to use ultrasound to coordinate performing procedures in real time. Some of the spatial reasoning questions will test your ability to:

- Identify what objects must be present but which you cannot see (hidden objects).
- Rotate three-dimensional structures to 'see' them from other perspectives.

In these question types it's easiest to assess each answer option in turn. Once you can eliminate an option, move on. You should then be left with one remaining correct answer.

Question 13

Below is a structure assembled from equally sized cubes. Which of the following options could represent the view of the structure from the top, side (as shown by the arrow) and front?

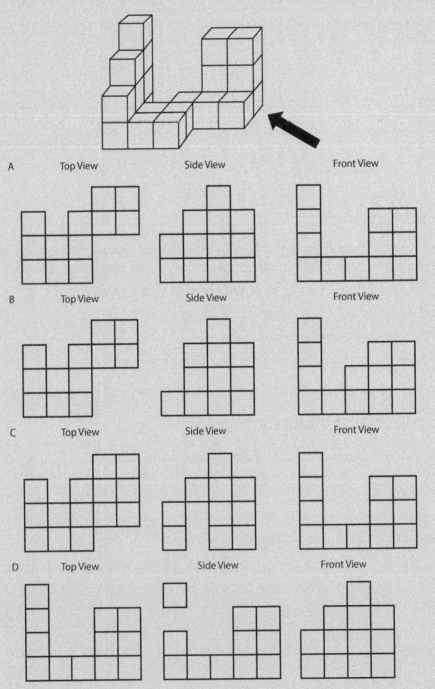

Question 13: answer and explanation

It is best to start with one side, and work your way through the answer options eliminating any which don't work. The easiest side to visualise is the front view, as you can almost see this in the diagram. By logically working your way through the options, eliminating them one by one, you are left with only one correct answer: A.

You could quickly have eliminated answer option D, as this features a 'floating' box in the side view. It would be physically impossible for the box to float above the structure, so this answer must be incorrect.

Construction and deconstruction

Assembly style questions require you to convert 2D shapes into 3D (or, on rare occasions, vice versa). Many students struggle with these questions, as they find it hard to visualise the transformation into three dimensions.

The easiest way to approach these questions is to:

1. Analyse each answer option in turn.

2. Start with one side (it's easiest to pick the largest).

3. Find the analogous area on the three-dimensional shape.

4. Compare the adjacent sides on the two- and three-dimensional shapes.

5. Eliminate combinations which don't match.

6. If two adjacent sides match, compare to the next adjacent side, etc.

7. Continue until you've eliminated all but one option.

Question 14

Which of the following boxes could be assembled from the shape below?

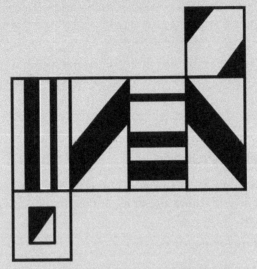

A.   B.   C.   D.   E. None of the below

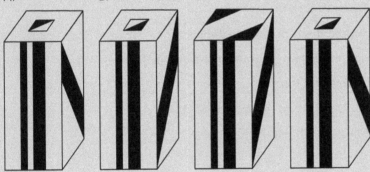

Question 14: answer and explanation

Using the above step-by-step approach, we can assess each answer option in turn. Starting with the largest side facing us and finding the analogous area on each of the two- and three-dimensional shapes, we can work through option by option:

A: The top and large faces do not match as the thick line should be on the same side as the black triangle, not the white triangle.

B: The large face and top work, but the diagonal stripe on the side should be angled such as in option A.

C: The top and large faces do not work as the triangles are positioned in the wrong corners.

D: Correct answer.

Navigation

Navigation questions test your ability to navigate an object through space. They can take a descriptive form or can present you with a three-dimensional shape which you need to move in a certain order through a grid. Questions will then focus on where the object will end up or which side will be visible.

These questions can be combined with basic geometry, although without a calculator you are unlikely to encounter questions involving π.

Top Tip: Questions can sometimes involve π where they will stipulate $\pi = 3$ to ensure calculations are possible without the use of a calculator.

The basic geometric formulae you need to know are covered in Section 2 – Maths.

Question 15

A dancer performs a dance that requires taking the following steps seven times:

- 5 steps forwards
- 5 steps to the right
- 2 steps backwards
- 1 step left

Each of the dancer's steps has a length of 40 cm.

What is the displacement, in metres, of the dancer from their original position at the end of the dance?

A. 5.2 m

B. 7 m

C. 10.4 m

D. 13 m

E. 14 m

Question 15: answer and explanation

A good way to approach this problem is to think in vectors. It may help to draw a diagram of the dancer's steps:

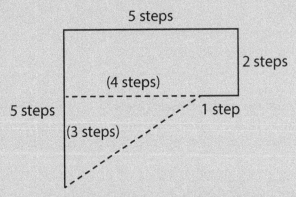

It is clear from the diagram that after each cycle the dancer has moved the vector equivalent of 3 steps forward and 4 steps to the right. Using Pythagoras' theorem, we can see that after one set of dance steps the dancer has moved: $\sqrt{3^2 + 4^2} = 5$ steps from their original position (alternatively you can quickly see this is a Pythagorean 3, 4, 5 triangle).

This happens 7 times, so they move 7 x 5 = 35 steps from their original position. Each step is 40 cm in length, so they are displaced by 35 x 0.4 = 14 m from their original position.

Top Section 1 Tips:

- Practise each question style in turn.
- Learn and understand the definitions and structure of an argument.
- Use the past papers on the BMAT website and the questions on The Medic Portal website.
- Practise questions to time.
- Get used to working without a calculator.

Overview

The second section of the BMAT exam is the science section. It requires scientific knowledge to GCSE (Key Stage 4) level in:

- Biology
- Chemistry
- Physics
- Maths

Although most students will be studying some or all of these subjects at a higher level, many still find this section challenging. This is because although the knowledge required is GCSE level, the *application* of the knowledge can require significant initiative and 'thinking outside the box'.

A BMAT syllabus (test specification) is available on the BMAT website. This lists all the topics and specific knowledge required. There is also an 'assumed knowledge guide' available on the BMAT website. This science revision guide can be read online but cannot be downloaded or printed.

Format of the section

Section 2 contains 27 multiple choice questions to be answered in 30 minutes. This equates to just over a minute per question. As per Section 1, you must answer the questions on the computer-read answer sheet provided using a pencil. If you mark more than one answer option per question, you will not score any points.

Top Tip: Every question is worth one mark and there is no negative marking. You should therefore never leave any answers blank – if in doubt try to eliminate answer options and make an educated guess.

Question format

There will be six to eight questions in each of chemistry, biology and physics, and five to seven in maths. There are slightly fewer maths questions as mathematical skills will already have been covered in Section 1. There is no set order of questions or topics.

We will now work through the BMAT syllabus for all four science subjects. At the end of the book there is a mock exam containing sample questions with model answers.

Biology

1. Cell biology

1.1 Cell structure

You should learn the names, locations and functions of the following cellular structures:

Animal cells

Structure	Function and other key details
Cell membrane	• Separates the internal and external environment of the cell • Regulates the movement of substances in to and out of the cell • Involved in cell-to-cell signalling • Composed of a phospholipid bilayer
Cell nucleus	• Contains nuclear DNA, in the form of chromosomes • Bound by nuclear membrane • Regulates the activities of the cell through transcription of DNA
Cytoplasm	• 'Gel-like' substance in cell where many enzyme-catalysed reactions take place, e.g. glycolysis
Ribosomes	• Protein and RNA structures that synthesise proteins • Site of translation
Mitochondrion (*pl.* mitochondria)	• Double membrane-bound structures that synthesise energy for the cell in the form of ATP • Also contains mitochondrial DNA and regulates its transcription

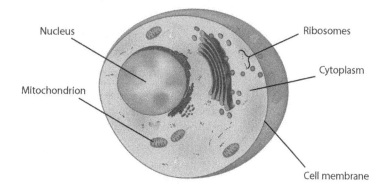

Plant cells

Plant cells have all the structures contained within animal cells as well as additional structures, including:

Structure	Function and other key details
Cell wall	• Rigid structure made from **cellulose** that maintains the shape of the cell and prevents it from bursting under osmotic pressure
Chloroplast	• Double membrane-bound structure that is the site of photosynthesis • Also contains chloroplast DNA and regulates its transcription
Permanent vacuole	• Contains sap, which draws in water by osmosis and maintains the cell's turgidity

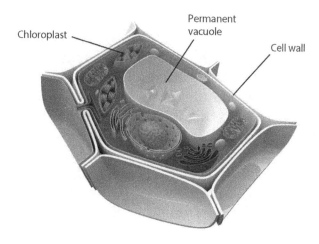

Bacterial cells

Bacterial cells *do not* contain a cell nucleus, mitochondria or chloroplasts, and other structures may differ significantly from corresponding structures in animal and plant cells:

Structure	Function and other key details
Cell wall	• Rigid structure made from **peptidoglycan** that maintains the shape of the cell and prevents it bursting under osmotic pressure
Nucleoid/Chromosomal DNA	• Large ring of DNA containing most of the cell's genetic material • It is free-floating in the cytoplasm, i.e. not bound by a membrane
Plasmid	• Small ring of free-floating DNA • May code for antibiotic resistance; the transfer of plasmids between bacterial cells helps spread resistance
Flagellum (*pl.* flagella)	• 'Whip-like' structure that is used for motility • Not found on all bacterial cells

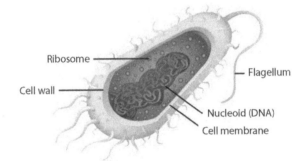

Ribosome

Cell wall

Flagellum

Nucleoid (DNA)

Cell membrane

Top Tip: It is very common in the BMAT to be asked whether a statement is true or false. Often, statements will be presented in a way such that they sound true when in fact they are false (and vice versa). A common way examiners do this is by writing a statement that is half-true, or even mostly true, but with a subtle error that renders the statement false as a whole. Since biology is, broadly speaking, a more descriptive subject than physics or chemistry, this type of 'trick' is very common in BMAT Biology questions (although it will be inevitably used in some questions for the other subjects too!). Consider this statement:

'The nucleoid is a structure found within bacterial cells consisting of a ring of membrane-bound DNA.' This is mostly correct, except of course for the fact that the nucleoid is *not* membrane bound. It may seem obvious, but similar statements in the BMAT are often subtler and easier to miss when you are under stress!

1.2 Movement across cell membranes and into cells

You need to know six ways in which substances can move across cell membranes:

1. **Diffusion:** The movement of dissolved particles from a region where they are highly concentrated to a region where they are less highly concentrated. Movement is *passive* and *down* a concentration gradient. Substances that move across cell membranes by diffusion must be nonpolar or small enough to dissolve directly into membrane (e.g. CO_2, O_2), or they require a protein channel in the membrane (also known as facilitated diffusion, e.g. glucose).

2. **Osmosis:** The movement of water across a semi-permeable membrane from a region of low solute concentration (or high water potential) to a region of high solute concentration (or low water potential). Movement is *passive* and *down* a concentration gradient (i.e. that of water).

3. **Active transport:** The movement of substances *against* a concentration gradient. This requires energy-consuming transport proteins in the membrane.

4. **Phagocytosis:** The movement of large particles into the cell by the infolding of a region of cell membrane.

5. **Pinocytosis:** The movement of liquid into the cell by the infolding of a region of cell membrane.

6. **Exocytosis:** The movement of substances out of the cell by the fusing of vesicles with the cell membrane.

1.3 Cell division and reproduction

Mitosis

This type of cell division produces the new cells that are needed for growth, replacement and repair. It produces somatic cells (non-gametes) and has the following steps in humans:

1. The chromosomes in the parent cell are duplicated. There are normally **23 chromosome pairs** in a human somatic cell.

2. The duplicated chromosomes line up at the centre of the cell.

3. The duplicated chromosomes are pulled apart at their centres (*centromeres*).

4. *Two* daughter cells form with exactly the same number of chromosomes as the parent cell, i.e. **23 pairs – 46 chromosomes**. They are *diploid* cells. The daughter cells are *genetically identical* to the parent cell.

Meiosis

This type of cell division produces gametes (sex cells – sperm, produced in the testes, and ova, produced in the ovaries). It leads to the production of genetically different gametes. It has the following steps:

1. The chromosomes in the parent cell are duplicated.

2. Chromosomes in the *same pair* line up and exchange sections of DNA by *crossing over*. This means that the chromosomes in each pair are no longer genetically identical.

3. Individual chromosomes in each *pair* are separated from each other.

4. The duplicated chromosomes are then pulled apart at their centres.

5. *Four* daughter cells are formed with half the number of chromosomes as the parent cell, i.e. **23 chromosomes**. They are *haploid* cells. The gametes that are produced are genetically different from the parent cell, and from each other.

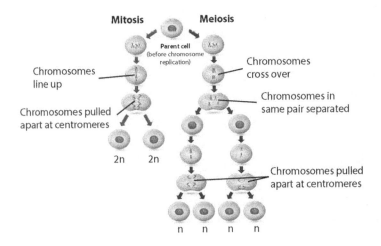

Asexual reproduction

This is when one parent produces offspring that are genetically identical (i.e. clones).

Sexual reproduction

This is when two parents produce offspring that are genetically different from both parents – since each parent contributes half of the offspring's chromosomes through their gametes, and these chromosomes may have undergone crossing-over during meiosis. It increases genetic variation in a population.

Sex determination

Sex in mammals is determined by the sex chromosomes, X and Y. Females have two X chromosomes (XX) and males have one X and one Y (XY). The expected sex ratio of offspring is 50:50 male to female, since there is a 50% chance that any individual will receive a Y chromosome from their father, and a 50% chance that they will receive an X chromosome.

Top Tip: Remember that during both mitosis *and* meiosis there is an initial doubling in the amount of genetic material within the cell as copies of *each chromosome* are made. Since we already have two chromosome copies in each cell, this means that before division we have the equivalent of *four* copies of each *chromatid* in each cell. Chromatids become new chromosomes. Remember also that *every* cell in the body, excluding the gametes, has the full complement of chromosomes – including sex chromosomes.

1.4 Enzymes

Enzymes are biological catalysts made from proteins. They speed up the rate of biological reactions without being used up themselves. An enzyme-catalysed reaction takes place in the enzyme's **active site**. Reactant molecules, or the **substrates**, fit into the active site because the active site has a specific shape.

If the shape of the active site is altered because of protein denaturation, the enzyme will become ineffective at catalysing the reaction.

Temperature and its effect on enzyme-catalysed reactions

As temperature increases, the rate of an enzyme-catalysed reaction will also increase as collisions between substrate articles and the enzyme active site become more likely. At the **optimum temperature** the rate of reaction is at it fastest. Above this temperature, the enzyme begins to denature and the rate of reaction falls sharply.

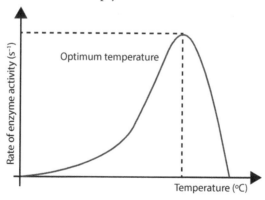

Graph showing how temperature affects the rate of an enzyme-catalysed reaction

pH and its effect on enzyme-catalysed reactions

The rate of an enzyme-catalysed reaction is fastest at a particular pH, the **optimum pH**. At pH values lower or higher than the optimum pH, the enzyme begins to denature and the rate of reaction falls sharply.

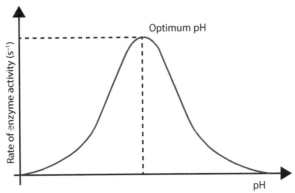

Graph showing how pH affects the rate of an enzyme-catalysed reaction

2. Genetics

2.1 Terminology

Gene: A section of DNA that codes for a particular protein.

Allele: Different forms of the same gene.

Genotype: A description of the alleles possessed by a particular organism.

Phenotype: A description of the physical characteristics of a particular organism.

Dominant: A characteristic that develops when the allele that codes for it is present on one or both chromosomes in a pair.

Recessive: A characteristic that *only* develops when the allele that codes for it is present on both chromosomes in a pair.

Homozygous: When an organism possesses the same allele on each chromosome in a pair.

Heterozygous: When an organism possesses different alleles on each chromosome in a pair.

2.2 Monohybrid crosses

Make sure you understand how Punnett squares work:

		Mother's alleles	
		A	a
Father's alleles	A	AA	Aa
	A	AA	Aa

They can be used to figure out the expected ratio of offspring genotypes from parent genotypes. For instance, in this example, a mother and a father with genotypes of Aa and AA respectively can be expected to produce 50% of offspring with genotype AA and 50% with Aa. Remember, an organism carrying a dominant allele for a trait *must* express that trait, regardless of whether it is heterozygous or homozygous. Recessive alleles will *only* be expressed in homozygous organisms.

Punnett squares can be used in conjunction with **genetic pedigrees** to work out the probability that an individual will display a particular trait and determine the pattern of inheritance. Remember, for pedigrees *usually* males are represented with squares and females are represented with circles. Individuals expressing the trait are shaded black and individuals not expressing the trait are left white.

Autosomal dominant traits (e.g. Huntington's disease)

- If just *one* parent is homozygous dominant, all offspring will express the trait.
- If one parent is heterozygous and expresses the trait and other parent does not express the trait, 50% of offspring will express the trait.
- If both parents are heterozygous then 75% of offspring will express the trait.
- Parents that do not express the trait do not transmit the trait.
- Appears in both sexes with equal frequency and both sexes can transmit the trait to their offspring.
- Does not tend to skip generations.

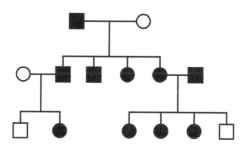

Autosomal recessive traits (e.g. cystic fibrosis)

- If *both* parents are homozygous recessive, all offspring will express the trait.
- If one parent is homozygous recessive and the other is heterozygous, 50% of offspring will express the trait.
- If both parents are heterozygous, 25% of offspring will express the trait.
- Parents that do not express the trait can produce offspring that express the trait.
- Appears in both sexes with equal frequency and both sexes can transmit to offspring.
- Trait may skip generations.

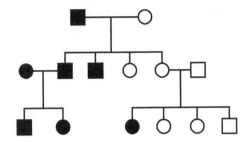

X-linked dominant traits (e.g. Rett syndrome)

- Both sexes express the trait but it tends to be more common in females than in males.
- Sons expressing the trait must also have a mother expressing the trait.
- Daughters expressing the trait must have a mother or a father expressing the trait.
- Fathers expressing the trait will pass it on to all their daughters, but cannot have sons with the trait.

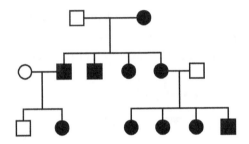

X-linked recessive traits (e.g. haemophilia)

- Both sexes affected but it tends to be more common in males than in females.
- Sons expressing the trait may be born to mothers not expressing the trait.
- It is never passed from father to son.

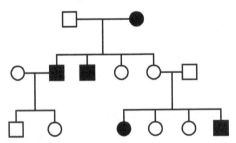

Y-linked dominant traits

- Only males affected; passed from fathers to sons.
- Does not skip generations.

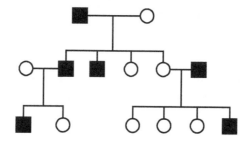

> **Top Tip:** Although we have given you some example pedigrees, remember that there is no 'set' pedigree for any type of inheritance. Learning these examples by heart will not help when you sit your exam. Instead, when given a pedigree, look at each generation in turn and ask yourself which inheritance patterns could have led to that particular expression profile? Work your way through the different branches of the pedigree and you should be able to narrow down the possible inheritance patterns until you come to a correct answer.

2.3 Genetic variation

Note that variation can be caused by the *environment* as well as one's genes. Many traits show variation due to both environment *and* genetics (e.g. weight, height). However, only genetic variation can be *inherited*. Genetic variation is caused by **crossing-over** during meiosis, **sexual reproduction** and **mutation**.

Genetic variation is vital to **evolution by natural selection**. Variation leads to organisms that show differing levels of adaptation to their environment; hence some organisms will be better at surviving than others. Organisms that survive are able to reproduce and pass on their adaptive traits to their offspring.

Continuous variation: The trait varies gradually over a range of values. If influenced predominantly by genetic variation, the trait is usually under the control of many genes (traits include height, weight, skin colour).

Discontinuous variation: The trait can be placed definitively into one of a small number of discrete categories. If influenced predominantly by genetic variation, the trait is usually under the control of a small number of genes (traits include gender, blood group).

3. DNA and gene technologies

3.1 DNA structure

Genes are made from deoxyribonucleic acid, or DNA. A DNA molecule consists of a **double helix** constructed from a sugar, deoxyribose, a phosphate and bases. The sequence of the four bases, adenine (A), thymine (T), cytosine (C) and guanine (G), determines the genetic code. Bases demonstrate **complementary pairing**: A pairs with T, G pairs with C.

In animal and plant cells, DNA is arranged in long strands wrapped around protein molecules to form **chromosomes**.

3.2 Protein synthesis

Proteins are made from **amino acids**. Triplets of bases in DNA code for different amino acids; the order of base triplets in DNA determines the order of amino acids in the protein.

Transcription is the first step in protein synthesis: a molecule of **mRNA** is transcribed from DNA by enzymes in the nucleus. The sequence of bases on the mRNA is determined by complementary pairing with bases on the DNA.

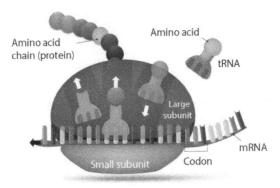

Translation follows: The strand of mRNA is passed through ribosomes in the cytoplasm. Molecules of **tRNA** also pass through the ribosome; each molecule of tRNA carries an amino acid molecule. Triplets of bases on the mRNA (known as **codons**) pair with complementary triplets on molecules of tRNA. The ribosome then joins together the amino acids carried by the tRNA to form a protein.

3.3 Mutations

Any alteration in the sequence of bases within DNA is called a mutation. Mutations can occur spontaneously, or they may be induced by **mutagens** such as tar from cigarette smoke or radiation. Mutations may not necessarily have an effect – they may occur in non-coding regions of DNA, for instance.

3.4 Gene technologies

Genetic modification: Using enzymes, genes can be cut from the DNA of one organism using a **restriction enzyme** – these enzymes cut DNA at *specific sites*. The desired gene is then placed into the DNA of another organism using a **ligase enzyme** which sticks DNA at specific sites. This means the second organism expresses a gene that it would not normally. Examples include the insertion of herbicide-resistance genes into crops and the insertion of the human insulin gene into bacteria (for the mass-production of insulin for diabetics).

Top Tip: When questions reference genetic modification, make sure you have a firm understanding of which type of chemical is used at which stage. For instance, it is *not* true that 'insulin is transferred into a bacterial vector' in the example above – insulin is a *protein*. Rather, it is the insulin *gene* that is transferred. It may seem obvious now, but often this type of subtle wording is used to trip up candidates.

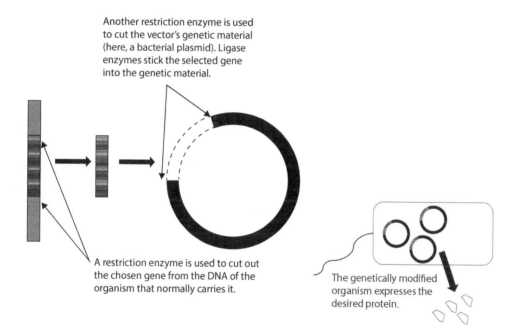

Another restriction enzyme is used to cut the vector's genetic material (here, a bacterial plasmid). Ligase enzymes stick the selected gene into the genetic material.

A restriction enzyme is used to cut out the chosen gene from the DNA of the organism that normally carries it.

The genetically modified organism expresses the desired protein.

3.5   Stem cells

Cells in the early embryo give rise to all the different cell types in the body. They are called **embryonic stem cells** and have the potential to differentiate into any cell type. As the embryo grows, cells become more and more specialised and lose the ability to do this. It may be possible to use embryonic stem cells therapeutically in tissues that do not self-repair easily, such as in the brain.

Stem cells may also be found in adult (non-embryonic) tissues. These **adult stem cells** can be found, for instance, in bone marrow. Although adult stem cells can differentiate into many types of cell they lack the ability possessed by embryonic stem cells to turn into *any* type of cell in the body.

4. Physiology

4.1 Nervous system

The nervous system consists of the **central nervous system (CNS)**, the brain and spinal cord, and the **peripheral nervous system**, a network of nerves that connect the limbs and organs with the central nervous system.

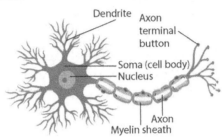

A neurone is a nerve cell; it receives signals from other neurones at its **dendrites** and passes on signals to other neurones via its **axon**. *Electrical* signals are passed along single neurones.

Chemical signals, called neurotransmitters, pass between neurones across a small gap called a **synapse**.

A **reflex arc** is the nerve pathway that is used during a **reflex action**. The signals in a reflex arc are transferred rapidly because they bypass the brain. They pass through the flowing sequence of neurones:

1. **Sensory neurones** transmit signals from **receptors** – specialised cells that detect certain stimuli (e.g. temperature, pressure etc.).

2. **Relay neurones** (also known as **interneurones**) are found in the CNS and transmit signals from sensory neurones to motor neurones; they regulate the flow of signals in the CNS.

3. **Motor neurones** transmit signals from relay neurones to **effectors**. They elicit a response by the effector. An effector is a specialised tissue that responds to a stimulus – it might be a gland or a muscle.

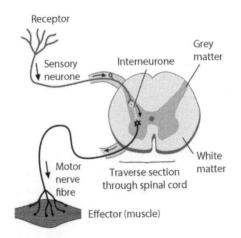

Top Tip: The brain is *not* involved in a reflex arc.

4.2   Respiratory system

Ventilation

Ventilation is the process whereby air is moved into and out of the lungs to allow for gas exchange. Airways bring air into the lungs: the **trachea** leads from the mouth and nose; its shape is maintained by **C-shaped rings of cartilage**. The trachea branches into two **bronchi** (*sing.* bronchus). These in turn branch into smaller **bronchioles**. The smallest bronchioles end with air sacs called **alveoli** (*sing.* alveolus) – these are the sites of gas exchange.

The lungs sit in a fluid-filled cavity called the **pleural cavity**. The pleural cavity is contained by two **pleural membranes**; these are slippery, to stop them from sticking to each other during breathing.

Breathing is controlled by the **diaphragm** (the muscular floor of the chest cavity) and the **inter-costal muscles** (the muscles between the ribs).

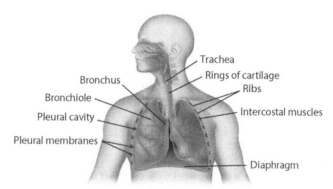

When we **inhale**, the diaphragm contracts and moves downwards. The *internal* intercostal muscles relax and the *external* intercostal muscles contract, causing the ribcage to move upwards and outwards. This increases the volume of the thoracic cavity and lowers the air pressure inside the cavity. Higher-pressure air from outside the cavity moves into the lungs so that air pressure is equilibrated. Air movement into the lungs causes them to inflate. Inhalation replenishes oxygen-rich air in the lungs so that alveolar gas exchange can occur.

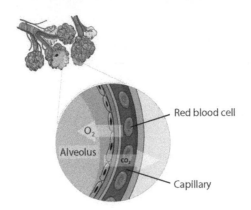

Red blood cell

O_2

Alveolus

CO_2

Capillary

When we **exhale**, the diaphragm relaxes and moves upwards (passive expiration). The *internal* intercostal muscles contract and the *external* intercostal muscles relax, causing the ribcage to move downwards and inwards (active expiration). The volume of the thoracic cavity is reduced, increasing air pressure in the cavity. Air moves out of the lungs so that air pressure is equilibrated. The lungs deflate. Exhalation removes CO_2-rich air from the lungs so that alveolar gas exchange can occur; it is also the primary mechanism of CO_2 excretion from the body.

Gas exchange

Gas exchange is what occurs in the lungs when gases are transferred between the **alveoli** and the blood of the alveolar circulation. Deoxygenated blood arriving in the lungs contains a high concentration of CO_2 relative to the alveolar air. It diffuses down its concentration gradient across the capillary and alveolar walls into the alveolus. Conversely, alveolar air contains a relatively high concentration of oxygen which diffuses into the blood where it combines with **haemoglobin** in red blood cells, forming **oxyhaemoglobin**.

> **Top Tip:** Haemoglobin without any bound oxygen is called deoxyhaemoglobin. Students often confuse this with carboxyhaemoglobin which is haemoglobin bound with carbon monoxide, not dioxide!

4.3 Respiration

Respiration is distinct from **breathing**; it is a process that occurs in *all* tissues and cells of the body. It describes the *chemical process* by which energy is released from nutrients.

Aerobic respiration is the process in which *oxygen* is reacted with *glucose* to produce *energy*. *Water* and *carbon dioxide* are also produced as waste products. It is a multi-step process that occurs partially within the cell's cytoplasm and partially within the mitochondria.

Glucose + Oxygen → Energy + Carbon Dioxide + Water

Anaerobic respiration is the incomplete breakdown of glucose to release energy in the absence of oxygen. In animal cells, the reaction also produces *lactic acid* or *lactate*, which causes cellular pH to drop. The body has to subsequently convert the lactic acid into CO_2 and water by reacting it with oxygen. Hence, during anaerobic respiration, an *oxygen debt* is built up.

$$Glucose \rightarrow Energy + Lactic\ Acid$$

4.4 Circulatory system

Humans have a *double* circulatory system; with each complete circuit of the body, blood passes through the heart *twice*. From the heart, blood undergoes two circuits, as follows.

Pulmonary circulation

Deoxygenated blood from the heart goes to the lungs via the *pulmonary artery*. The blood is under lower pressure than in the systemic circuit. It passes through capillaries that surround the alveoli. The blood becomes oxygenated through gas exchange – the newly oxygenated blood is returned to the heart via the *pulmonary vein*.

Systemic circulation

Oxygenated blood is sent to the rest of the body – initially by passing through the *aorta*. The blood is pumped under high pressure to maintain a good flow rate around the body. It passes from arteries to arterioles, and from here it goes through capillaries. Every cell in the body is close enough to a capillary such that it receives all the oxygen it needs through diffusion alone. Deoxygenated blood from the tissues returns back to the heart through venules and veins; it enters the heart via the *venae cavae*.

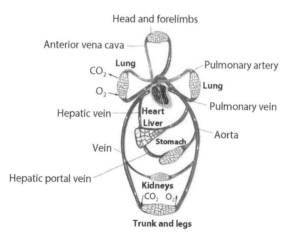

> **Top Tip:** The pulmonary arteries and veins are exceptions to the rule: the pulmonary artery carries deoxygenated blood while the pulmonary vein carries oxygenated blood.

The heart

The heart is a muscular organ that pumps blood around the body. It is made from *cardiac muscle*, a type of involuntary muscle that can generate its own contraction. *Deoxygenated* blood enters the heart on the *right* side, via the superior and inferior *venae cavae*. It first enters the *right atrium*, which then pumps the blood through the *tricuspid valve* to the adjacent *right ventricle*. The right ventricle then pumps blood into the *pulmonary artery* through the *pulmonary valve*.

Oxygenated blood enters the heart on the left-hand side via the *pulmonary vein*. It first enters the *left atrium*, which then pumps the blood through the *bicuspid* or *mitral valve* to the *left ventricle*. The *left ventricle* then pumps blood into the *aorta* through the *aortic valve*. The wall of the *left* ventricle is thicker than the wall of the right ventricle, reflecting the fact that the right ventricle pumps blood with more force to maintain a high systemic circulatory pressure.

The heart itself is supplied with oxygenated blood via the *coronary arteries*. If these become blocked, the cardiac muscle lacks oxygen and may die – this is a myocardial infarction (heart attack).

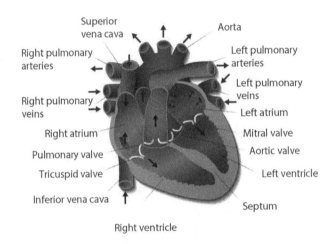

Top Tip: Make sure you have a very good understanding of circulation, both within the body and the heart. It is common to get trick questions along the lines of 'Is this statement true – the vena cava transports deoxygenated blood from the body into the left atrium'. The statement is *mostly* true, except of course the vena cava delivers blood into the *right* atrium. As always with the BMAT, pay close attention to the wording and read the question carefully.

Blood vessels

Arteries carry blood away from the heart. They tend to carry oxygenated blood; an exception is the *pulmonary artery*. They have thick walls relative to their lumen – this is because the walls contain smooth muscle and elastic tissue to resist and maintain high pressure of blood that has just been pumped from the heart.

Veins carry blood towards the heart. They tend to carry deoxygenated blood; an exception is the *pulmonary vein*. Veins tend to carry blood at a lower pressure, as it has already passed through the capillary network. Hence, veins have relatively large lumens relative to their vessel walls. In addition, because they carry blood at relatively low pressure, they often contain *one-way valves* to prevent the backflow of blood.

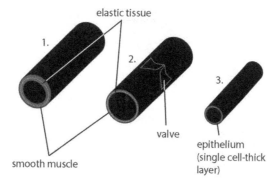

Capillaries are narrow blood vessels. They have vessel walls that are one cell thick – this aids gas exchange with surrounding tissues by reducing the distance over which gases have to diffuse.

4.5 Digestive system

Food enters the **alimentary canal** through the **mouth**, which begins digestion by chewing and mixing the food with saliva produced by the **salivary glands**. Saliva contains **salivary amylase**.

From the mouth, food passes through the **oesophagus**, a muscular tube which utilises **peristalsis** to move the food into the **stomach**. The stomach uses muscular contraction to break down the food; it also produces **protease** enzymes. Protease has a low optimal pH, so the stomach also produces **stomach acid**. Stomach acid has the added advantage of killing pathogens, thereby forming part of the innate immune system.

From the stomach, the food passes into the **duodenum** – the first section of the small intestine. Here, food is mixed with enzymes produced by the pancreas – **pancreatic amylase, protease and lipase**. The food is also mixed with **bile** – this substance is *synthesised* in the **liver**, but *stored* and *secreted* by the **gall bladder**. Bile has two roles: it emulsifies fats (making them easier to digest), and neutralises stomach acid, because it is alkaline.

From the duodenum, digested food (**chyme**) passes into the **jejunum** and the **ileum** – the second and third parts of the small intestine. They absorb nutrients from the digested food into the blood. Both the jejunum and the ileum have a large surface area to aid this absorption process – this is due to their length and the presence of **villi** on their inner surface.

What remains after digestion and absorption passes into the large intestine. The **colon** absorbs water; the **rectum** stores faeces, and the **anus** is the area from which faeces are egested.

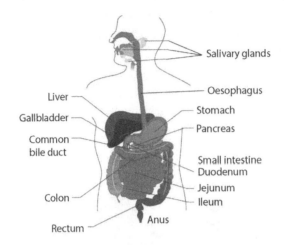

Digestive enzymes

Name of enzyme	Catalysed reaction	Produced by
Amylase	Starch into maltose	Salivary glands, pancreas
Maltase	Maltose into glucose	Small intestine
Lipase	Fat into glycerol and fatty acids	Pancreas, small intestine
Protease	Proteins into amino acids	Stomach, pancreas, small intestine

Peristalsis

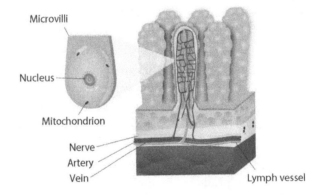

Peristalsis moves food along parts of the alimentary canal – it describes a synchronised contraction of smooth muscle in parts of the alimentary canal, such as the oesophagus and the small intestine. Contraction of *circular* smooth muscle causes the lumen to constrict; contraction of *longitudinal* smooth muscle causes localised shortening of the gut. The contractions progress in wave-like motions to 'push' food along.

Villi

Villi (*sing.* villus) are the protrusions found on the inner surface of the small intestine – they are adapted to absorb nutrients into the blood:

- They are coated with **microvilli** which increase their surface area; microvilli have a wall which is just one cell thick, minimising diffusion distance.
- Their surface is coated with digestive enzymes, such as maltase.
- They are well-supplied with capillaries, which carry nutrients away in blood.
- They contain a structure called a **lacteal** which transports fatty acids and glycerol away in the lymph.

Hepatic portal vein

This vessel transports blood from the small intestine to the liver. The liver helps to regulate the levels of certain nutrients in the blood (e.g. it turns excess glucose into glycogen and breaks down excess amino acids).

4.6 Renal system

The **kidneys** have an important role in excretion – they produce urine. Urine contains *excess water*, *urea* (a toxin produced in the breakdown of amino acids) and some *excess salts*. Urine is passed from the kidneys through the ureters to the **bladder**, where it is stored. It then leaves the bladder, and the body, through the **urethra**.

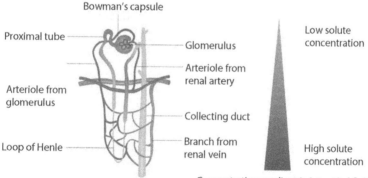

Bowman's capsule
Proximal tube
Glomerulus
Arteriole from renal artery
Arteriole from glomerulus
Collecting duct
Loop of Henle
Branch from renal vein
Low solute concentration
High solute concentration
Concentration gradient in interstital fluid

Microscopic structures called **nephrons** are found within the kidneys – they regulate the water content of the blood that passes through the kidneys. Each nephron is in close association with blood capillaries.

The first part of the nephron is the **Bowman's capsule**. It surrounds the **glomerulus**, a network of capillaries. Blood enters these capillaries under high pressure – this forces water, toxins (including urea), amino acids, sugar and salt out of the capillaries. This process is called **ultrafiltration**. Proteins are too large to be filtered, and remain in the blood.

The filtrate is collected by the Bowman's capsule. It passes into the next section of the nephron – the **proximal convoluted tubule**, where glucose, amino acids and some salt are reabsorbed into the blood via active transport.

Then the fluid passes into a structure called the **Loop of Henle**. Here, reabsorption of water and salt establishes a concentration gradient in the **interstitial fluid** surrounding the nephron. The fluid leaving the loop is *dilute*.

This dilute fluid then passes into the **collecting duct**. The water content of the fluid in the collecting duct can be altered depending on the permeability of the collecting duct to water. When the duct is highly permeable, water moves into the **interstitial fluid** by osmosis. The permeability of the duct is regulated by **antidiuretic hormone (ADH – see below)**. Fluid leaving the collecting duct is called urine.

4.7 Homeostasis

Homeostasis is the maintenance of a constant internal environment within narrow limits, independent of external factors. Homeostasis is usually maintained through **negative feedback** mechanisms – whereby any change in the internal environment is detected and countered with a response that *reverses* that change.

Thermoregulation

Thermoregulation is how the body maintains a constant internal temperature of around 37°C. It is controlled by the **hypothalamus** in the brain, which detects the temperature of blood. The hypothalamus elicits different responses in the body if the internal temperature drops or rises too much.

Internal temperature	Hairs on skin	Sweat	Capillaries in the skin	Skeletal muscles
Too hot	Flatten	Is secreted onto skin by sweat glands; heat is lost as the sweat evaporates.	Vasodilation – more blood is brought to the surface of the skin, where it loses heat by radiation.	Shivering does not occur.
Too cold	Are erected by the contraction of small muscles within the skin; this traps a layer of insulating air close to the skin.	Is not secreted	Vasoconstriction – less blood is brought to the surface of the skin; instead it flows beneath insulating layers of subcutaneous fat.	Shivering occurs – this generates heat

Osmoregulation

Osmoregulation is how the body maintains the osmolarity of fluids. The osmolarity of blood is monitored by the hypothalamus. This, in turn, regulates the amount of ADH released by the **pituitary gland** in the brain.

When blood is **too dilute**, ADH release from the pituitary gland is *reduced*. Water filtered from the blood in the kidneys (see above) leaves the body as urine. Dilute urine is produced.

When the blood is **too concentrated** with solutes, ADH production from the pituitary is *increased*. Higher levels of ADH in the blood cause the permeability of the collecting ducts in the kidney to increase. More water leaves the collecting duct by osmosis and is reabsorbed in the kidney. Concentrated urine is produced.

Top Tip: Remember, higher levels of ADH in the blood leads to less urine being produced.

Blood glucose regulation

Blood glucose regulation maintains relatively constant concentrations of glucose within the blood. Glucose levels are detected by cells in the pancreas. When glucose levels are *too high*, β–**cells** within the pancreas secrete **insulin** into the blood. When glucose levels are *too low*, α–**cells** within the pancreas secrete **glucagon** into the blood. Insulin and glucagon are hormones with opposing effects in the body:

Effects of...	On the liver	On fat tissue
Insulin	Promotes the uptake of glucose by the liver and its conversion within the liver to glycogen.	Promotes the uptake of glucose by fat tissue and its conversion into lipids.
Glucagon	Promotes the breakdown of glycogen into glucose and its release into the blood.	Promotes the breakdown of lipid.

Top Tip: Use the mnemonic: alpha cells produce glucagon when the glucose in your blood has 'gone'.

4.8 Hormones

Hormones are chemicals that are used to regulate processes in the body by providing a (relatively) long-lasting signal that travels in the blood. They are released from **endocrine glands** – these, by definition, release hormones *directly* into the blood. They are distinct from **exocrine glands** which do *not* release hormones, but release other substances (e.g. bile, sweat) into a cavity or outside the body via a *duct*.

As well as the hormones already described, you should be aware of the hormones that regulate the **menstrual cycle**:

Hormone	Released from...	Physiological effect	Effect on other hormones
Follicle stimulating hormone (FSH)	Pituitary gland	Matures the egg in the ovary, within a *follicle*.	*Promotes* the production of **oestrogen** by the ovaries
Oestrogen	Ovaries	Causes thickening of the uterine wall	*Inhibits* release of **FSH**, hence its use in contraceptive pills. Causes a 'surge' in **LH**.
Luteinising hormone (LH)	Pituitary gland	Causes the release of the mature egg from the *follicle* (ovulation)	Causes **progesterone** to be produced by the ovaries.
Progesterone	Ovaries – specifically the *corpus luteum*, what remains of the follicle after ovulation	Maintains the uterine wall. If the egg is not fertilised, progesterone levels drop and this causes the uterine wall to break down.	*Inhibits* the production of **FSH** and **LH**, thus preventing the release of two eggs at once.

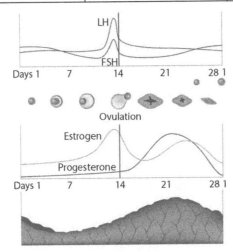

You should also be aware of these other hormones (note the additional role of oestrogen):

Hormone	Released from...	Physiological effect
Adrenaline	Adrenal glands	Varied, including: • Increased heart rate • Increased metabolism • Redirection of blood to muscles • Expansion of airways
Testosterone	Testes	Male sexual characteristics
Oestrogen	Ovary	Female sexual characteristics

4.9 Immune system

Innate immunity describes the general defences that the body has against infection, of any sort. It consists of physical barriers such as the skin, mucous membranes, stomach acid, etc. In addition, specialised white blood cells called **phagocytes** can identify, attack and consume microbes that invade the body.

Acquired immunity describes the body's ability to form a more rapid defensive response to microbes that it has previously encountered. Key to this response is two other types of white blood cell:

- **B-cells**, which produce **antibodies**.
- **T-cells**, which produce **antitoxins** and can kill infected cells of the body.

Antibodies are proteins that recognise and bind to molecules (*antigens*) on the cell surface of a previously encountered pathogen. They immobilise the pathogen, clump microbes together and help phagocytes to consume them.

5. Environment

5.1 Food chains and populations

In food chains, energy moves from food to the animal feeding on that food. Plants are known as **producers** in the food chain, because they are able to capture energy from the sun via photosynthesis. Producers are consumed by **primary consumers**, who are consumed by **secondary consumers**, and so on.

At each stage of the food chain, some energy is lost to the surroundings as *heat* or in the form of waste *materials*.

Apart from these losses to the surroundings, the food that animals eat will be converted into living material, or biomass. The amount of biomass is decreased at each stage of the food chain because:

- there are energy losses to the surroundings at each stage of the food chain
- not all the biomass at one stage of the food chain will be consumed by organisms at the next stage of the food chain.

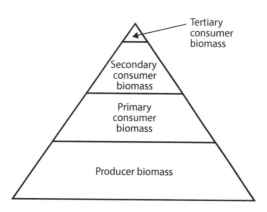

This causes the shape of a 'biomass pyramid'.

You need to be aware that **populations** of organisms interact with each other. The predator–prey relationship is one example of such an interaction. Note that changes in the population of one organism can have 'knock-on' effects on the population of another organism. Hence, in predator–prey relationships, populations may follow cyclical patterns as a decreasing prey population leads to a decreasing predator population, which in turn causes the prey population to increase, and so on.

5.2 Carbon cycle

Carbon dioxide enters the **atmosphere** by three main routes:

a) **Respiration** of organisms – producers, consumers and decomposers.

b) **Combustion** of organic material or fossil fuels.

c) **Weathering** of carbonate-containing rocks (e.g. limestone) and **volcanic activity**.

Carbon is assimilated into **organisms** by three main routes:

a) **Producers** (plants) extract carbon from carbon dioxide in the air and convert it into glucose during **photosynthesis**.

b) **Consumers** acquire their carbon by eating plants, and by eating other consumers.

c) **Decomposers** acquire their carbon by breaking down dead organisms, or the waste of living organisms.

Carbon may accumulate **elsewhere** in the environment:

a) If decomposition is prevented, carbon from dead organisms may turn into **fossil fuels**.

b) Many marine animals create shells from **calcium carbonate**. Over time, their shells may become **carbonate-rich minerals**, such as limestone.

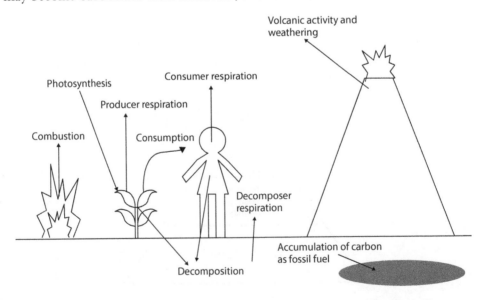

5.3   Nitrogen cycle

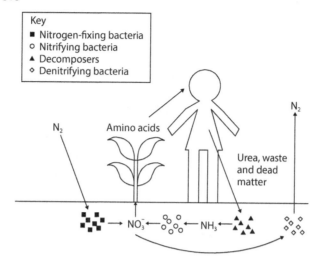

Key
- ■ Nitrogen-fixing bacteria
- ○ Nitrifying bacteria
- ▲ Decomposers
- ◇ Denitrifying bacteria

Nitrogen gas is present in high quantities in the air. It is converted into **nitrate** by **nitrogen-fixing bacteria** and **lightning**. **Nitrifying bacteria** convert **ammonia** into **nitrates**. **Plants** absorb nitrates and convert them into **amino acids**. These are then passed on to **consumers**. **Urea**, **egested material** and **dead organisms** are broken down by **decomposers**, which returns nitrogen to the soil as **ammonia**. **Denitrifying bacteria** break down **nitrates** into **nitrogen gas**, which is released into the atmosphere.

Chemistry

1. The atom

1.1 Atomic structure

An atom is a small unit of matter. It is composed of three even smaller particles:

- **Neutrons** have a relative atomic mass of 1. They are not charged.
- **Protons** have a relative atomic mass of 1. They have a positive charge.
- **Electrons** have negligible atomic mass. They have a negative charge.

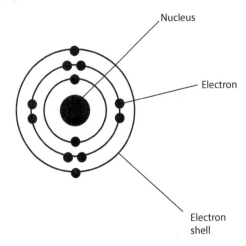

The atom consists of a central **nucleus**, which contains protons and neutrons clustered together. Electrons orbit the nucleus; they can only follow orbital paths at set distances from the nucleus. The orbits that they occupy are called **electron shells**. The shell *closest* to the nucleus can hold a maximum of two electrons. Shells further out can hold a maximum of eight electrons.

In an atom, the numbers of electrons and protons are equal, so the atom has no overall charge.

Atoms may, however, lose or gain electrons to become **ions**. Ions have an overall charge that is positive (if electrons are lost) or negative (if electrons are gained). A positive ion is known as a **cation**, a negative ion is an **anion**.

The **relative atomic mass** (A_r) of an atom is given as the sum of the total number of protons and neutrons it contains.

The **atomic number** of an atom is equal to the total number of protons it contains. The atomic number differentiates atoms of different elements.

Standard notation shows the chemical symbol of an element, as well as its mass number (in superscript, before the symbol) and its atomic number (in subscript, before the symbol), e.g. $^{12}_{6}C$ for carbon.

The atomic number can be used to write an electronic configuration, which tells us the number of electrons in each shell. For example, as carbon has an atomic number of six, there must be six protons and six electrons in each atom. Its electronic configuration is {2, 4}. Similarly, the atomic number of calcium is 20, so it has an electronic configuration of {2, 8, 8, 2}. You only need to know how to write electronic configurations for the elements from hydrogen to calcium.

The mass of a molecule, in terms of atomic mass, is the sum of all the individual masses of *each* atom that makes up the molecule. This is termed the **relative molecular mass (M_r)**. The M_r of ethane, C_2H_6, is therefore equal to the mass of two carbon atoms and six hydrogen atoms $= (2 \times 12) + (6 \times 1) = 30$.

1.2 Isotopes

The isotopes of an element refer to atoms of that element that have *different masses* but have the *same* atomic number. That is, they each have the same number of *protons* but different numbers of *neutrons*.

In the periodic table, the relative atomic mass of each element is given as a *weighted average* of all the atomic masses of the different isotopes of that element, depending on how common they are.

To work out the relative atomic mass of an element, sum the atomic mass of each isotope multiplied by its relative abundance (as a percentage). For instance, neon has three naturally occurring isotopes: ^{20}Ne, ^{21}Ne and ^{22}Ne, with relative abundances of 90.5%, 0.25% and 9.25% respectively. So its relative atomic mass is: $(20 \times 0.905) + (21 \times 0.0025) + (22 \times 0.0925) \approx 20.18$

1.3 Chemical bonding

Single atoms will react with other atoms in order to gain a **full outer shell** of electrons, or, in other words, to gain the electronic configuration of a **noble gas** (see below).

Atoms of the *same* element may bond together, e.g. in molecules of O_2 and N_2. Atoms of *different* elements may also bond together to produce **compounds**.

There are three types of bonding that you need to be aware of:

- **Covalent bonding**: a covalent bond consists of a *pair* of electrons that is shared between two atoms. One electron in each pair may be provided by each bonded atom, or both electrons may be provided by a single atom – the bond in the latter case is known as a **dative bond**. Covalent bonds tend to form between atoms of *non-metal* elements.
- **Ionic bonding**: atoms may *lose* or *gain* electrons from their outer electron shell in order to attain a noble gas configuration. When electrons are lost or gained, the overall charge on the atom changes – the atom becomes an **ion**. Ionic bonds occur due to the natural affinity that ions of opposite charges will have for each other (i.e. a positive ion will be strongly attracted to a negative ion). Ionic bonding tends to occur between atoms of *metallic* elements and *non-metallic* elements.
- **Metallic bonding**: the outermost electrons of metal atoms can become dissociated from their atoms. This results in a *system* of dissociated electrons around metal cations. The bonding is due to the affinity of the positive cations to the negative dissociated electrons.

You also need to be aware of four molecular structures that come about as a result of this bonding:

- **Simple covalent structures**: these consist of a few atoms held together by *strong* covalent bonds. They have *weak* intermolecular forces, so these molecules tend to have low melting and boiling points. Examples include CO_2, H_2O, NH_3, O_2 and N_2.

- **Giant covalent structures**: these consist of a large number of atoms joined together by covalent bonds to form **giant, repeating lattice structures**. Since the structure is held together by strong covalent bonds, they tend to have very high melting and boiling points. You need to know the identities of several giant covalent structures:

  - **Silica**: consists of a lattice of oxygen and silicon atoms; each silicon atom is bonded to four oxygen atoms and each oxygen atom is bonded to two silicon atoms. It is hard with a high melting point, and is an electrical semiconductor.

  - **Graphite**: is an **allotrope** of carbon (i.e. one type of molecular arrangement of carbon). It consists of *layers* of carbon atoms arranged in lattice 'sheets'. A system of dissociated electrons exist between the layers; these electrons can transfer heat and carry an electrical current, so graphite is a good heat and electrical conductor. While the bonding between atoms *within* a layer is strong, the bonding *between* layers is fairly weak. Hence layers can slide over each other, making graphite fairly soft.

  - **Diamond**: is another allotrope of carbon. It is arranged such that each carbon atom is bonded to four other carbon atoms. It is extremely hard, with very high melting and boiling points. However, unlike graphite, it does not have dissociated electrons so it is a poor conductor of electricity.

- **Ionic lattice structures**: ions will arrange themselves into repeating lattice structures in which positive ions are surrounded by negative ions and negative ions are surrounded by positive ions. Due to the strong electrostatic forces holding the ions of different charges together, these structures have high melting and boiling points. As solids, they are poor electrical conductors, but when molten or dissolved in solution the ions are free to move about and can carry a current.

- **Giant metallic structure**: Layers of metal cations surrounded by dissociated electrons. The electrons carry heat and current, and so metals are good thermal and electrical conductors. The attraction between the cations and the electrons means that the structure tends to be strong, with high melting and boiling points. The cation layers can slide over each other, however, making metals malleable and ductile.

2. The Periodic Table

The Periodic Table displays **groups** (columns) of elements and **periods** (rows). For the BMAT, you should know that elements of the same *group* have the same number of outer-shell electrons, and elements of the same *period* have the same number of electron shells.

Elements in the same *group* tend to share similar chemical properties.

The elements in the periodic table can be divided into **metals** and **non-metals**. Their positions are displayed below. Down a *metal* group, reactivity increases; down a *non-metal* group, reactivity decreases.

1	2	3	4	5	6	7	8	9	10	11	12	13	14	15	16	17	18
H																	He
Li	Be											B	C	N	O	F	Ne
Na	Mg											Al	Si	P	S	Cl	Ar
K	Ca	Sc	Ti	V	Cr	Mn	Fe	Co	Ni	Cu	Zn	Ga	Ge	As	Se	Br	Kr
Rb	Sr	Y	Zr	Nb	Mo	Tc	Ru	Rh	Pd	Ag	Cd	In	Sn	Sb	Te	I	Xe
Cs	Ba	57-71	Hf	Ta	W	Re	Os	Ir	Pt	Au	Hg	Tl	Pb	Bi	Po	At	Rn
Fr	Ra	88-103	Rf	Db	Sg	Bh	Hs	Mt	Ds	Rg	Cn	Uut	Fi	Uu	Uu	Uus	Uu

La	Ce	Pr	Nd	Pm	Sm	Eu	Gd	Tb	Dy	Ho	Er	Tm	Yb	Lu
Ac	Th	Pa	U	Np	Pu	Am	Cm	Bk	Cf	Es	Fm	Md	No	Lr

The Periodic Table of Elements

2.1 Metals

Metals tend to be *ductile* (they can be stretched to form wires), *malleable* (they can be bent), and good conductors of *heat* and *electricity*. Certain metals have specific properties, which makes them useful for specific tasks:

- Aluminium: good strength-to-weight ratio, used in aircraft.
- Titanium: good strength-to-weight ratio, used in replacement hips, military aircraft.
- Iron: pure iron is a relatively soft metal, but iron with a certain carbon content forms *steel*, which is strong and used in construction.
- Copper: does not react readily with water, so it is used in pipes. Soft and easily bent, so used in wiring.
- Gold, silver, platinum: unreactive, but expensive; used in jewellery. Gold is a good conductor of electricity and is used in wires and circuits as it doesn't corrode.

2.2 Metal extraction

Metals are not usually found in their elemental state in nature, but are mined as **ores**. These are usually metal oxides. Metals are extracted when the metal oxides are *reduced*. Different metals require different extraction methods.

Reactive metals, such as potassium, sodium, calcium, magnesium and aluminium have to be extracted by *electrolysis* (see below).

Iron is less reactive than carbon, so it can be *displaced* by carbon.

Copper can also be extracted by being reacted with carbon. It is then purified by electrolysis.

Metals such as gold are so unreactive that they are found in their elemental state in nature.

2.3 Metals and displacement reactions

Metals have different levels of **reactivity**. When a more reactive metal is reacted with a less reactive metal that is in a compound with another element, the more reactive metal can **displace** the less reactive metal from the compound. For example, iron displacing less reactive copper from copper sulfate:

iron + copper sulfate → iron sulfate + copper

The relative reactivities of different metals is illustrated below. Certain non-metal elements (in italics) have also been included for reference:

Potassium

Sodium

Lithium

Calcium

Magnesium

Aluminium

Carbon

Zinc

Iron

Hydrogen

Copper

Silver

Gold

Top Tip: Learn this displacement table by heart! You will not be provided with it when you sit your BMAT, unlike your GCSE chemistry exams!

2.4 Alkali metals

Group 1 of the periodic table contains the **alkali metals**. They share similar properties:

- They are soft enough to be cut with a knife.
- They have low melting and boiling points relative to other metals.

- They have low densities (lithium, potassium and sodium float on water).
- They react violently with water to produce hydrogen and a metal hydroxide.
- Their hydroxides and oxides dissolve readily in water to produce alkaline solutions, hence their name.

As you descend the group, the Group 1 metals become *softer*, have *decreasing* melting points, *higher* densities, and they become *more reactive*.

The Group 1 metals are *so* reactive that they need to be kept under oil to prevent them from oxidising rapidly, but also to prevent a violent reaction with moisture in the air.

You need to know how Group 1 metals react with different substances:

- With **water**: Metals will react to form the metal hydroxide and hydrogen gas.

$$X_{(s)} + H_2O_{(l)} \rightarrow XOH_{(aq)} + H_{2(g)}$$

Lithium, sodium and potassium will all float on water. Potassium will produce a lilac flame during this reaction.

- With **oxygen**: Metals will react with air to form a layer of the metal oxide:

$$4X_{(s)} + O_{2(g)} \rightarrow 2X_2O_{(s)}$$

When *burned* in oxygen, lithium will react to produce lithium oxide (Li_2O). Sodium will produce *some* sodium oxide (Na_2O) *and* some sodium peroxide (Na_2O_2). Potassium, when burned, will form mostly potassium peroxide (K_2O_2). Lithium burns with a red flame, sodium with an orange flame and potassium with a lilac flame.

- With **halogens**: The metals react violently with the halogens to form a metal halide. For example, with chlorine:

$$2X_{(s)} + Cl_{2(g)} \rightarrow 2XCl_{(s)}$$

2.5 Transition metals

The transition metals are found in between Groups 2 and 3 (also written as Group 13) on the periodic table. They share similar properties:

- They form coloured compounds, e.g. copper (II) sulfate is blue, iron (III) oxide is red.
- They tend to be less reactive than Group 1 metals.
- They can have more than one stable ion, or *oxidation state*, e.g. iron can exist in compounds as a +2 or a +3 iron (these are the most common, but it can form others).
- They are often used as *catalysts*, e.g. iron is used in the reaction forming ammonia from nitrogen and hydrogen; nickel is a catalyst for hydrogenation.
- They tend to be strong, malleable, good conductors of heat and electricity, and have high densities.

2.6 Halogens

The halogens are the non-metal elements found in Group 7 (or Group 17). They share similar properties:

- They react vigorously with the alkali metals.
- Low melting and boiling points (typical of non-metals).

The reactivity of the halogens *decreases* down the group. The melting/boiling points *increase* down the group – fluorine and chlorine are both gases at room temperature, bromine is an orange liquid and iodine is a grey solid (that *sublimes* into a purple gas when heated).

More reactive halogens further up the group can *displace* less reactive halogens further down the group. You need to know how to write the *ionic equations* that describe this process; e.g. the displacement of chlorine by fluorine can be represented by:

$$2Cl^-_{(aq)} + F_{2(g)} \rightarrow Cl_{2(g)} + 2F^-_{(aq)}$$

The presence of different halide *ions* in solution can be tested using silver nitrate solution. First, dilute nitric acid is added to the solution to remove any carbonates that are present (as these would produce a precipitate of silver nitrate that would interfere with the results). Then silver nitrate is added:

- If a **white** precipitate is formed that dissolves with the addition of *dilute* ammonia solution, the solution contains **chloride** ions.
- If a **cream** precipitate is produced that dissolves in *concentrated* ammonia solution, the solution contains **bromide** ions.
- If a **yellow** precipitate is formed that does *not* dissolve in concentrated ammonia solution, the solution contains **iodide** ions.

2.7 Noble gases

The noble gases are the non-metal elements found in Group 8/0 (or Group 18). They share similar properties:

- They are very unreactive because they have a full outer electron shell.
- Under standard conditions, they are gases made up of *single atoms* of the element (i.e. unlike oxygen, O_2, or nitrogen, N_2, for example).
- They have low densities – helium is used in air balloons for this reason.

Because they are so unreactive, the noble gases are often used to prevent other reactions from happening. For instance, argon is used in light bulbs to prevent the filament reacting with air and burning.

3. Chemical reactions and equations

In a chemical reaction, the atoms within different compounds are *rearranged* but matter is *never* created or destroyed. The mass of reactants will always be equal to the mass of products.

A chemical reaction can be displayed as an **equation**. The equation can either be expressed in words or with **chemical symbols**. The state of different reactants and products may also be shown using **state symbols** – (s) for solid, (l) for liquid, (g) for gas and (aq) for a substance in aqueous solution.

Be aware of the symbols for these commonly used chemicals:

Hydrogen, H_2	Carbon dioxide, CO_2	Sulfuric acid, H_2SO_4
Oxygen, O_2	Water, H_2O	Hydrochloric acid, HCl
Nitrogen, N_2	Ammonia, NH_3	Nitric acid, HNO_3
Carbon monoxide, CO	Caustic soda	
	(Sodium hydroxide), NaOH	

You also need to be able to recall the charge on common ions. Note that the positive charge on metal ions will be the same as their group number in the periodic table. Transition metals, which form more than one stable ion, will have the charge of their ion indicated by Roman numerals, e.g. the ion of iron (III) is Fe^{3+}.

Ammonium, NH_4^+	Fluoride, F^-	Hydroxide, OH^-
Hydrogen, H^+	Chloride, Cl^-	Oxide, O^{2-}
Silver, Ag^+	Bromide, Br^-	Sulfide, S^{2-}
Lead, Pb^{2+}	Iodide, I^-	Sulfate, SO_4^{2-}
Carbonate, CO_3^{2-}	Nitrate, NO_3^-	Hydrogen carbonate, HCO_3^-

3.1 Balancing equations

Since mass is always conserved during a chemical reaction, the number of atoms of reactants in a chemical equation must equal the number of atoms of products.

Chemical equations therefore need to be *balanced* before they are correct.

The best way to approach balancing equations is perhaps to reduce it to an algebraic problem.

For example, with the equation:

$$PCl_5 + H_2O \rightarrow H_3PO_4 + HCl$$

We can put in the letters a, b, c, d and e to represent the balancing numbers:

$$aPCl_5 + bH_2O \rightarrow cH_3PO_4 + dHCl$$

We know that:

$a = c$ (from looking at the number of phosphorus atoms)

$5a = d$ (from looking at the number of chlorine atoms)

$2b = 3c + d = 3c + 5a$ (from looking at the hydrogen atoms)

$b = 4c$ (from looking at the oxygen atoms)

Let $a = 1$

$b = 4$

$c = 1$

$d = 5$

These are all whole numbers, so the balanced equation is:

$$PCl_5 + 4H_2O \rightarrow H_3PO_4 + 5HCl$$

Of course, if the letters happened to be *fractions* after substituting a for 1, you would have to multiply throughout by the *lowest factor* that would leave whole numbers to end up with the correct balancing numbers.

3.2   Redox reactions

When atoms of an element *gain* electrons as a result of a reaction, they are said to be **reduced**.

When atoms of an element *lose* electrons as a result of a reaction, they are said to be **oxidised**.

A **disproportionation** reaction is one in which atoms of the same element are both oxidised *and* reduced. When reduction and oxidation occur in the same reaction (but not necessarily to the same element), that is a **redox** reaction.

Note that, at a basic level, oxidation is defined as the gain of oxygen and reduction is the loss of oxygen.

> **Top Tip:** Remember the mnemonic OILRIG (Oxidation Is Loss, Reduction Is Gain).

Although you should not have to solve complicated ionic equations in your exam, it may be worthwhile to learn the following rules about oxidation states:

- The *overall* oxidation number of an uncharged compound should be zero.
- Group 1 metals always have an oxidation number of +1.
- Group 2 metals always have an oxidation number of +2.
- The oxidation numbers of elements in compound ions (e.g. NO_3^-, SO_4^{2-} etc.) must sum to the charge on the ion.

- Oxygen is *usually* −2, except in hydrogen peroxide, H_2O_2, where it is −1 (and F_2O where it is +2).
- Hydrogen is *usually* +1, except in the metal hydrides where it is −1.
- Chlorine is *usually* −1, except in compounds with oxygen and fluorine.
- Fluorine is *always* −1.

To work out balanced redox equations, first write out balanced *half-equations* for each species that is being oxidised/reduced. Then combine these half-equations to form a full, balanced equation. For example, the reaction describing the displacement of copper from copper (II) oxide by magnesium can be described with two half-equations:

$$Cu^{2+} + 2e^- \rightarrow Cu$$

and

$$Mg \rightarrow Mg^{2+} + 2e^-$$

Giving us an ionic equation of

$$Mg + Cu^{2+} \rightarrow Mg^{2+} + Cu$$

3.3 Reversible reactions

Sometimes, the products of one reaction can react themselves to form the original reactants. Such reactions are called **reversible reactions**.

Sometimes a reversible reaction may be in **dynamic equilibrium** whereby the rate at which the products are produced is the same rate at which products react to form the original reactants. Hence the amount of reactants and products remains constant, even though a chemical reaction is always occurring.

An example of such a reaction is the reaction of nitrogen with hydrogen to form ammonia:

$$N_2 + 3H_2 \rightleftharpoons 2NH_3$$

The forward reaction is exothermic and the reverse reaction is endothermic. For all reversible reactions, the **position of equilibrium** (i.e. how much reactant there is in relation to the amount of product) can be altered by two factors:

- **Temperature**: cooler temperatures will push the point of equilibrium towards the *exothermic* side of the reaction; hotter temperatures will push it to the endothermic side.
- **Pressure**: higher pressures will push the point of equilibrium towards the side of the reaction with *fewer moles of gas*; lower pressures will favour the side with *more moles of gas*.

Note that if a large quantity of reactants is suddenly introduced to a reaction system, the forward reaction will be favoured until the previous point of equilibrium has been re-established (provided that pressure and temperature have not changed). If large amounts of products are suddenly introduced to the system, the reverse reaction will be favoured.

Note also that catalysts have *no* effect on the position of equilibrium. They increase the rate of the forward and reverse reactions *to the same extent*, which may mean that a point of dynamic equilibrium is reached *faster* than it would without the catalyst.

4. Quantitative chemistry

4.1 The mole

A **mole** is simply a large number. Specifically, if you have one mole of any substance, the mass of that substance will be equal to its relative molecular mass (or relative atomic mass if we are considering pure elements) expressed in grams. So one mole of carbon (A_r = 12) has a mass of 12 g.

From this, we get the equation:

$$\text{number of moles in a sample of a subtance} = \frac{\text{mass of subtance}}{\text{relative molecular (or atomic) mass}}$$

Or

$$moles = mass/M_r$$

Using this equation, you may be asked to:

- Work out the **empirical formula** of a reaction (i.e. the formula that shows the simplest *proportions* of atoms involved in a reaction), based on the experimental masses of reactants and products. To do this, work out the number of moles of each reactant and product. Then find the ratio of the number of moles of each substance.
- Work out the **molecular formula** (i.e. the formula that shows the *total* number of atoms reacting with each other) using the empirical formula and M_r values. For instance, if I am looking at a reaction involving a hydrocarbon that is shown to be CH in my empirical formula, and if I then find out the M_r of my hydrocarbon is 26, I must have two lots of carbon and hydrogen atoms, since the M_r of CH would be 13. Hence the hydrocarbon in my molecular formula will be C_2H_2.
- Use **balanced equations** to calculate the masses of reactants and products. In a simple reaction X → 2Y + Z, if I have 0.1 moles of X (worked out from the mass of X), I must have 0.2 moles of Y (from this, I can work out my mass of Y) and one mole of Z.
- Calculate the **percentage composition by mass** of a compound given A_r values. If I know a sample of a compound has a certain mass, I can work out the number of moles of each element within the compound using the A_r values and the chemical equation for that substance, and subsequently work out the mass of each element. For instance, if I have a 23 g gram sample of ethanol (C_2H_5OH, A_r values: C = 12, O = 16, H = 1) and

I am asked to work out the percentage carbon by mass, I know that 1 mole of ethanol has a mass of 46 g, so I must have half a mole of ethanol in the sample. Hence I have one mole of carbon in the sample, which must be contributing 12 g to the total mass. So its percentage carbon by mass is 12/23 or ~ 52%.

4.2 Moles and gases

You will be told in the exam that 1 mole of any gas occupies 24 dm³ at room temperature and pressure (20°C and 1 atmosphere), and 22.4 dm³ at standard temperature and pressure (0°C and 1 atmosphere). From this you may be asked to work out the mass, the number of moles or the volume of gas.

Top Tip: Pay close attention to whether the question refers to *room* or *standard* conditions.

4.3 Moles and concentration

Using the equations

$$concentration\ (moldm^{-3}) = \frac{moles}{volume\ (dm^3)}$$

and

$$moles = \frac{volume\ (cm^3)}{1000} \times concentration\ (moldm^{-3})$$

you will be expected to work out moles, volume and concentration. You are also expected to work out the *solubility* of a substance in a particular solvent, i.e. how many moles of a given substance will dissolve in a given volume of solvent under certain conditions. Solubility can be expressed as a concentration.

Note that, at a given temperature and pressure, a solute will only dissolve into solution up to a certain point. Once a solution has become **saturated**, any further solute that is added to the solution will form a precipitate. The saturation point can be altered by changing the temperature and pressure of a solution.

4.4 Yield

You need to be able to work out the percentage yield of a reaction according to this equation:

$$percentage\ yield = \frac{actual\ yield\ (g)}{predicted\ yield\ (g)} \times 100\%$$

where predicted yield is obtained using a balanced equation, the mole equation, and the known masses of reactants.

Note that, in real life, when you measure the amount of products that can be usefully employed, the predicted yield is never obtained. This may be because of:

- unreacted reactants in a reversible reaction
- reactants that react in an unexpected way
- reactants left in their transfer containers (e.g. droplets left on the inside of flasks)
- products left inside reaction vessel.

5. Separation techniques

There are procedures that can separate the components of both mixtures (not chemically joined, but substances mixed together) and compounds (chemically bonded substances).

5.1 Miscible liquids

A mixture of liquids that are **miscible**, i.e. one does not float on top of the other when mixed, can be separated in several ways, including:

- **Chromatography**: separating substances depending on how well they dissolve in, or move through, another medium. A typical example is **paper chromatography**, where different inks can be separated depending on their solubility in water (and hence how far they are carried by water that is absorbed by a piece of filter paper).
- **Fractional distillation**: Different liquids in a mixture will have different boiling/condensing points. If these liquids are heated together, and if the gases that are evolved are passed through a **fractionating column**, the substance with the *higher* boiling point will condense first and can be collected separately. This method is used to separate the different components of crude oil (see diagram below).

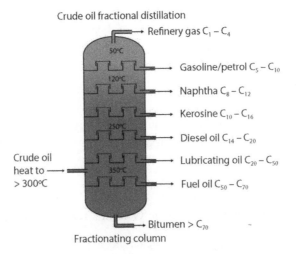

Crude oil fractional distillation

5.2 Immiscible liquids

Liquids that form separate layers when mixed can easily be separated by removing them one at a time with a **separating funnel**.

5.3 Soluble solids mixed with insoluble solids

These can be separated by **dissolving** the soluble solid in a solvent to form a solution that can be easily removed. The solution can be **filtered** to remove impurities. The liquid can then be **evaporated**, leaving the **crystallised** soluble solid.

5.4 Separating compounds – electrolysis

The components of certain compounds may be separated using **displacement reactions**; using a more reactive substance to 'push out' one element in a compound.

Electrolysis is a process that is used to separate out the component elements of ionic-bonded substances that have been melted or dissolved in solution. Such substances are called **electrolytes**. During electrolysis, a positive electrode, known as an **anode**, and a negative electrode, known as a **cathode**, are placed in an electrolyte. **Cations** in the electrolyte are attracted to the **cathode**, where they are *reduced*. Conversely, **anions** are attracted to the **anode**, where they are *oxidised*.

For electrolysis to work, a DC current has to be applied instead of an AC current, otherwise the polarity of the electrodes would keep switching.

You need to know about the electrolysis of the following substances:

Brine: When a solution of sodium chloride (NaCl) is electrolysed, **chlorine** gas is produced as chloride ions are oxidised at the **anode**:

$$2Cl^-_{(aq)} \rightarrow Cl_{2(g)} + 2e^-$$

Hydrogen ions from the water are reduced at the **cathode** to form **hydrogen gas**:

$$2H^+_{(aq)} + 2e^- \rightarrow H_{2(g)}$$

Sodium ions are *more reactive* than hydrogen ions, so they stay in solution with **hydroxide ions** from the water. Hence, the products of this electrolysis are chlorine, hydrogen and sodium hydroxide (or caustic soda) solution.

In industry, this electrolysis is carried out using an **ion exchange membrane** to keep the hydroxide and chloride ions separated. The membrane is permeable to sodium ions, so sodium hydroxide can be extracted from one side.

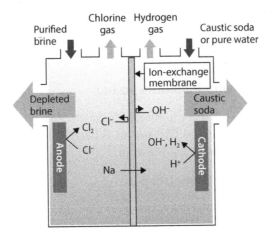

Copper (II) sulfate: This method can be used to purify impure copper. An **anode** of *impure* copper is used; at the anode, **copper (II) ions** are produced:

$$Cu_{(s)} \rightarrow Cu^{2+}_{(aq)} + 2e^-$$

These ions dissolve into solution. **Copper (II) ions** in solution are attracted to the **cathode** where they are *reduced* to form **pure copper** metal:

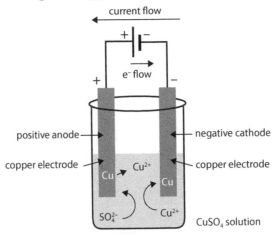

$$Cu^{2+}_{(aq)} + 2e^- \rightarrow Cu_{(s)}$$

6. Rates of reaction and energetics

6.1 Finding rates of reaction

Rates of reaction can be determined experimentally by measuring how quickly **a reactant is lost** or **a product is gained**. This might be done by using a **balance** to determine how quickly **mass is gained or depleted** if your reactants or products are liquids or solids. If your reactants or products are gases, you may be able to use equipment such as a **gas syringe** or a **measuring cylinder** to determine how quickly gas **volume is gained or depleted**.

You may also use **colorimetry** to determine how quickly a reaction progresses by measuring the change in light passing through the reacting chemicals (this can be done using a **colorimeter**).

You might also measure the rate of change of *properties* of the reacting chemicals, such as **electrical conductance** (which can be determined by observing changes in current using an **ammeter**), or **thermal conductance** (which can be measured using a **thermometer**).

6.2 Collision theory

For a reaction between different reactant particles to occur, two things must happen:

- The reactant particles must **collide**.
- The reactant particles must have a sufficient amount of energy when they collide, known as the **activation energy (E_A)**.

Collision theory explains why certain changes to the experimental environment can change the rate of reaction:

- **Changes in temperature**: If the temperature of a reacting system is *increased*, the reactant particles will have *greater* kinetic energy, and will be moving about faster (for this to be true, at least one of the reactants has to be in a fluid phase). This will *increase* the chance of collision between reactant particles, but it will also mean that when particles do collide, they are more likely to possess E_A. The reverse is true when temperature is *decreased*.
- **Changes in surface area**: If reactant particles are made more accessible by increasing the **surface area** of, for instance, a solid reactant (e.g. by grinding a block of the reactant into a powder), you increase the chance of a collision occurring.
- **Changing concentration**: If you increase the concentration of reactants in solution, or the partial pressures of gaseous reactants, you increase the likelihood of collisions occurring between reactant particles as there will be a greater number of the reactant particles in a certain volume.
- **Changing pressure**: Increasing the pressure of gaseous reactants will, again, increase the number of reactant particles in a given unit of volume, thereby increasing the chances of collisions occurring.

6.3 Rates of reaction graphs

Rates of reaction can be displayed *graphically*, usually by recording the **mass of reactant lost** or **mass of product gained** on the *y*-axis and **time** on the *x*-axis. Usually the line of the graph with be diagonal and straight initially (i.e. near the origin), but will plateau over time. See below.

Usually it is helpful to compare the *initial* rate of reaction under different conditions; that is, finding out the gradient of the straight line close to the origin. A *faster* initial rate of reaction will be shown with a *steeper* line (i.e. one with a *larger* gradient). A reaction with a faster initial rate will plateau earlier.

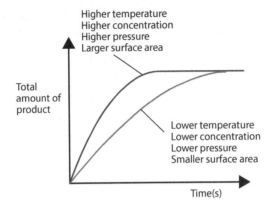

Note that by comparing the initial rate of reaction for different *concentrations* of a particular reactant, you can draw a **rate–concentration** graph; this allows you to establish the **order** of the reaction.

> **Top Tip:** When working out rate of a reaction from a graph similar to the one above, always use the *initial* rate, i.e. the region of the line that is *straight*.

6.4 Catalysts and energetics

All reactions require energy input in order to take place – this is the **activation energy**. This energy, ultimately, is required to break the bonds in the reactant molecules. When different bonds are formed in the products, energy is released.

If more energy is required to *break* bonds than is released by the formation of bonds, energy in the form of heat will be withdrawn from the environment as the reaction proceeds. Such reactions are known as **endothermic** reactions. Below is the energy profile for an endothermic reaction:

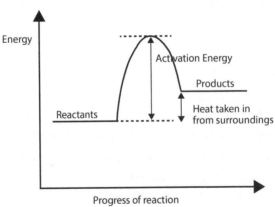

If more energy is released by the *formation* of bonds in the products than is required to break the bonds in the reactants, energy in the form of heat will be released into the environment as the reaction proceeds. Such reactions are known as **exothermic** reactions. Below is an energy profile for an exothermic reaction:

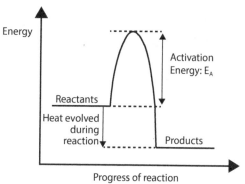

Catalysts are substances that *increase* the rate of a particular reaction, without being used up in the reaction themselves. They do this by *lowering* the activation energy required to initiate the reaction. An energy profile comparing catalysed and non-catalysed reactions is shown below:

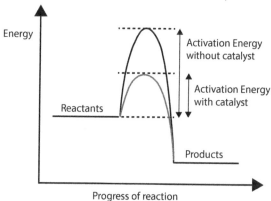

7. Acids and bases

An **acid** is a substance that releases **hydrogen ions** when dissolved in solution (it is a **proton donor**). A **strong acid** is one that fully dissociates to form hydrogen ions in solution whereas a **weak acid** does not fully dissociate. A **base** is a substance that neutralises acids (it is a **proton acceptor**). It usually does this by forming **hydroxide ions** when it is dissolved in water.

A **strong base** is one that is fully dissociated into its ions and produces a lot of hydroxide ions when in solution; a **weak base** does not dissociate fully and will result in a lower hydroxide concentration when in solution.

Acids have a pH **below** 7, bases have a pH **above** 7, and pH 7 itself is **neutral**.

> **Top Tip:** Examiners may try to trip you up by subtly referencing pH. For instance, you may be asked: 'Is this statement true? – Sodium hydroxide is a base, and will dissolve in water to form an alkaline solution with a low pH.' This is *mostly* correct, except of course that the pH will be *high* if the solution is alkaline.

Acids react with **bases** to form a **salt** and **water**, e.g.

$$HCl_{(aq)} + NaOH_{(aq)} \rightarrow NaCl_{(aq)} + H_2O_{(l)}$$

Acids react with **metals** to form a **salt** and **hydrogen**, e.g.

$$2HCl_{(aq)} + Mg_{(s)} \rightarrow MgCl_{2(aq)} + H_{2(g)}$$

Acids react with **carbonates** to form a **salt, water** and **carbon dioxide**, e.g.

$$2HCl_{(aq)} + CaCO_{3(s)} \rightarrow CaCl_{2(aq)} + H_2O_{(l)} + CO_{2(l)}$$

8. Organic chemistry

You need to know how to name hydrocarbon molecules according to International Union of Pure and Applied Chemistry (IUPAC) guidelines. The way to do this is as follows:

- Identify the longest carbon chain in the molecule; this will determine the 'root' of the hydrocarbon name to be used. For instance, if the longest chain is just 1 carbon, the root is 'meth'; 2 carbons, 'eth'; 3 carbons, 'prop'; 4 carbons, 'but'; 5 carbons, 'pent', etc.
- Identify the functional groups. The position of the main functional group is indicated by the number of the carbon atom that forms part of it or attaches to it. The number that is assigned to that carbon atom has to be the *lowest* number possible (given how far along the carbon chain it is). The functional group is indicated with a suffix or a prefix.
- Side chains are then identified. The position of the side chains is indicated by the number of the carbon atom in the main carbon chain to which they are attached.
- If there is more than one of the same side chain, the prefixes 'di' and 'tri' are used to indicate two or three of the same side chain, respectively.
- Side chains are named in alphabetical order (ignoring the 'di' and 'tri' prefix). Hence 'ethyl' will always precede 'methyl' in the full name of the hydrocarbon.

As an example, look at the molecule below:

- The longest carbon chain is 4 atoms long, so the root is 'but'.
- The molecule is an alkene; the lowest number carbon atom we could assign to establish the position of the alkene functional group is 1 (because the functional group is right at the end of the carbon chain). Hence we are looking at a 'but-1-ene'.
- There are two side chains with 1 carbon atom each, hence we have two methyl groups; so we need to add the prefix 'dimethyl'.
- They are both on carbon 3, so the full name is '3,3 – dimethylbut-1-ene'.

You need to know about the following types of hydrocarbon molecule:

Alkanes: C—C

- These hydrocarbons have a general formula of C_nH_{2n+2}
- They only contain *single* carbon–carbon bonds; hence we say that they are **saturated**.
- They are relatively unreactive, because the carbon–hydrogen and carbon–carbon bonds they contain are very stable.
- They can be **combusted** completely in excess oxygen to form water and carbon dioxide.
- They are indicated by the suffix 'ane'.

Alkenes: C=C

- Have a general formula of C_nH_{2n}
- They contain at least one *double* carbon–carbon bond; hence we say that they are **unsaturated**.
- We can **test** for alkenes by shaking them with **bromine water**; if an alkene is present, the bromine water will decolourise from orange.
- Alkenes are more reactive than alkanes because the carbon–carbon double bond can 'open up' to form single bonds with other atoms (i.e. alkenes are susceptible to addition reactions). You need to know about the following reactions:
  - **Hydrogen** – when alkenes react with hydrogen they form alkanes. The process is known as **hydrogenation**, and requires a nickel catalyst when carried out industrially. Here is the reaction of ethene with hydrogen:

$$C_2H_{4(g)} + H_{2(g)} \rightarrow C_2H_{6(l)}$$

- **Halogens** – alkenes will react with halogens to form dihaloalkanes. The carbon atoms that were previously in the double bond still have a single bond with each other, but they also each have a single bond to the halogen atom. Note that this *isn't* true for fluorine. Here is the reaction of ethene with chlorine:

$$C_2H_4 + Cl_2 \rightarrow C_2H_4Cl_2$$

- **Hydrogen halides** – alkenes will react with halogen halides to form haloalkanes. When an *asymmetrical* alkene is used, the halogen atom will *tend* to attach to the carbon atom in the carbon–carbon double bond that has the *fewest* hydrogen atoms already attached to it (you do not need to know why this is the case). Hence, in the reaction between propene and hydrogen chloride we get 2-chloropropane:

$$C_3H_6 + HCl \rightarrow C_3H_7Cl$$

- **Steam** – alkenes reacted with steam will produce **alcohols**. When steam is reacted with an asymmetrical alkene, the alcohol functional group (O H) will *tend* be added to the carbon atom in the carbon–carbon double bond that has the *fewest* hydrogen atoms already attached to it. Hence in the reaction between propene and steam we get propan-2-ol:

$$C_3H_6 + H_2O \rightarrow C_3H_7OH$$

Alcohols: O—H

- Alcohols tend to have higher melting and boiling points than their corresponding alkanes due to the presence of their −OH group, which permits **hydrogen bonding** between molecules.

- In addition, due to their −OH group they are soluble in water. They are also soluble in hydrophobic substances due to their hydrocarbon chains. Longer-chain alcohols are less soluble in water than shorter-chain alcohols.

- Alcohols can be used as fuels, as they burn easily in oxygen. Because they can be produced through the fermentation of biomass, they may be considered to be more eco-friendly than other fuels (as their combustion simply releases CO_2 that was taken up by the plant).

Carboxylic Acids

- Carboxylic acids are hydrocarbons with the functional group −COOH.
- When dissolved in water, these hydrocarbons form acidic solutions. They tend to form *weak* acids.
- Like all acids, they react with carbonates to form a salt, water and carbon dioxide. For example, the reaction of ethanoic acid with calcium carbonate to form calcium ethanoate:

$$CH_3COOH_{(aq)} + CaCO_{3(s)} \rightarrow CH_3COOCa_{(aq)} + H_2O_{(l)} + CO_{2(g)}$$

- They react with alcohols, in the presence of an acid catalyst, to form **esters** and **water**. For instance, ethanol reacts with ethanoic acid to form ethyl ethanoate:

$$C_2H_5OH_{(l)} + CH_3COOH_{(aq)} \rightarrow CH_3COOC_2H_{5(aq)} + H_2O_{(l)}$$

Polymers

Alkenes, or any organic molecule with a carbon–carbon double bond, can react with each other to form long, saturated molecules called polymers.

The unsaturated, simple molecules that join to create polymers are called **monomers**.

As an example, ethene can act as a monomer that can be polymerised to form **polythene**:

Most polymers are **non-biodegradable**, because micro-organisms lack the molecular machinery to break them down. Instead, they have to be disposed of by other means; for example, by being placed in landfills or incinerated. Both of these methods have detrimental ecological impacts.

Alternatively, some polymers are designed to be biodegradable. It is also possible to recycle many polymers.

Physics

1. Electricity

1.1 Electrostatics

A material may be an electrical **conductor**, in which case it will easily *disperse* any electrical charge that it gathers. Other materials may be electrical **insulators** that do not disperse charge easily.

If an insulator is rubbed it may become positively charged by *losing* electrons, or it may become negatively charged by *gaining* electrons. Friction causes the displacement of electrons.

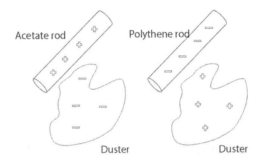

For instance, an **acetate** rod that is rubbed with a duster will lose electrons to the duster and become *positively* charged. A **polythene** rod that is rubbed with a duster will acquire electrons and become *negatively* charged (the duster will be positively charged).

Charged objects with the *same* charge will be repelled from each other. Objects with *different* charges will be attracted to each other.

Static electricity is useful in some cases in industry, e.g. it can be used in spray painting. The object that needs to be painted is given a particular charge, and the paint droplets are given the opposite charge as they are released. This means the paint is attracted to the object and less is wasted.

Static electricity also poses a danger in some cases. Build-ups of charge may eventually be dissipated in the form of a spark. In certain scenarios, such a spark may ignite a fire. Hence certain precautions need to be taken, for instance, with vehicles that are used to transport flammable substances. Any charge that is built up as the vehicle travels needs to be discharged using an earth wire – this reduces the chance of a spark igniting a fire.

1.2 Electric current

Current (I) is the flow of charge (usually electrons, although currents can be carried by other charged particles such as ions) through an electrical conductor. Its unit is the **ampere (A)**, which is the same as a coulomb (a measure of charge) per second. Hence it can be described by the equation:

$$\text{current (A)} = \frac{\text{charge (C)}}{\text{time (s)}}$$

Voltage (V) or **potential difference** is the work that needs to be done to move a unit of charge between two points. Without a potential difference across an electrical component, electrons will not flow through it and there will be no current. The unit of voltage is the **volt (V)**, which is equal to a joule per coulomb. It can be described by this equation:

$$\text{voltage (V)} = \frac{\text{work done (J)}}{\text{charge (C)}}$$

Current in a circuit is measured with an **ammeter**. An ammeter is always placed **in series** with other components in the circuit. Voltage is measured with a **voltmeter**; this device measures the potential difference across a single component in an electric circuit. In order to do so, it is placed **in parallel** to the component.

Resistance (R) describes the opposition to current in a conductor. All conductors have resistance. Resistance is *directly* proportional to the *length* of a wire but *inversely* proportional to the *cross-sectional area* of a wire. Resistance is measured in **ohms (Ω)**.

Voltage, current and resistance are all linked by this equation:

$$\text{voltage} = \text{current} \times \text{resistance}$$

or

$$V = IR$$

1.3   Voltage–current graphs

The relationship between voltage and current can be expressed graphically, with current on the *y*-axis and voltage on the *x*-axis.

In a **fixed resistor**, the resistance is maintained at a constant level. The current flowing through the resistor is *directly proportional* to the voltage across the resistor. Hence the graph is a straight, diagonal line.

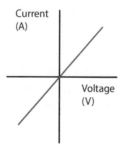

In a **filament lamp**, the filament heats up as more current passes through it. The heat that is generated increases the resistance of the filament. This means that resistance does not remain constant for all values of current, but will increase as current rises. This gives the graph a *sigmoidal* shape.

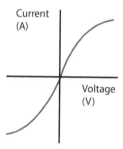

1.4   Series and parallel circuits

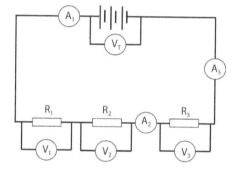

In a **series circuit**, components are placed in a 'loop' such that the same current passes through all components.

The **voltage** that is supplied to a series circuit (i.e. the voltage across the battery or cell) is equal to the **sum of the voltages across all components** in the circuit.

$$V_{tot} = V_1 + V_2 + V_3...$$

The **current** in series circuits is the same *wherever* it is recorded in the circuit.

$$I_1 = I_2 = I_3...$$

The **resistance** of the circuit is equal to the **sum of the resistances of all the components** in the circuit.

$$R_{tot} = R_1 + R_2 + R_3...$$

In a series circuit the total of all the resistors multiplied by the current taken at any point in the circuit will give you the voltage across the battery or cell, the **'voltage drop'**.

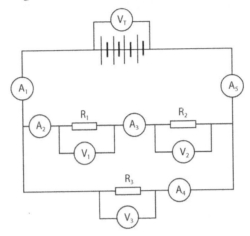

In a **parallel circuit**, components will not necessarily be connected one after another, but some components will be placed on parallel branches.

The **voltage** across components that are *arranged in parallel* is equal. In other words, the *sum* of the voltages across components on the same *branch* of a parallel circuit will equal the voltage across the battery or cell (i.e. in the diagram above $V_1 + V_2 = V_3 = V_T$).

The **current** entering and leaving a branching point in a parallel circuit must be equal. Hence, when several branches meet, the current after the meeting point is equal to the sum of the currents across each branch (in the diagram above $I_1 = I_2 + I_4 = I_5$).

Note that current recorded at any point on a *single* branch will always be the same, because current will not 'split' if there are no branch points – hence $I_2 = I_3$.

Bear in mind that, unlike voltage, the current on two different branches arranged in parallel is not necessarily equal. Hence, in the above example, it is not necessarily the case that $I_2 = I_4$.

The total **resistance** in a parallel circuit is given by the *reciprocal law*:

$$1/R_{tot} = 1/R_1 + 1/R_2 + 1/R_3...$$

Sometimes the circuits you are given in the BMAT exam will look very different from the easy-to-categorise series and parallel circuits you get at GCSE. For instance, have a look at this one:

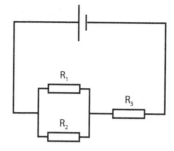

Is this a series or parallel circuit? In situations like this, it is better to consider the *arrangement* of components. Resistors R_1 and R_2 are arranged in parallel, so it may be easier to consider them as a 'single' resistor where the total resistance can be figured out from $1/R_T = 1/R_1 + 1/R_2$ (reciprocal rule!). After doing that, you are left with a much less scary-looking series circuit:

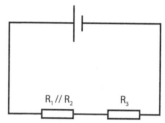

1.5 Electrical power

Power (P) is the rate of energy transfer, measured in **watts (W)**. A watt is equal to a joule per second. The transfer of electrical power can be given as:

$$power\ (W) = voltage\ (V) \times current\ (A)$$

Following on from this, the energy transfer in a component in an electrical circuit is

$$energy\ transfer\ (J) = power\ (W) \times time\ (s)$$
$$= voltage\ (V) \times current\ (A) \times time\ (s)$$

1.6 Transformers

Transformers are devices that allow **voltage and current** to be altered. Electricity produced by power stations needs to have its current reduced and its voltage increased when it is put into the National Grid, in order to prevent energy loss as heat in pylon cables. This requires a **step-up transformer**.

When electricity is sent to our homes, the voltage needs to be decreased and the current increased, for reasons of safety. This is carried out by **step-down transformers**.

A transformer consists of a **primary coil** wound round a **core**. Current flowing through the primary coil creates a magnetic field which then induces a current in a **secondary coil**. Alterations in current and voltage between the coils depend on the **number of turns** in both the primary and secondary coils. The transformer equation is given by:

$$\frac{\text{number of turns in primary coil}}{\text{number of turns in secondary coil}} = \frac{\text{voltage in primary coil (V)}}{\text{voltage in secondary coil (V)}}$$

Transformers are supposed to maintain electrical power while altering voltage and current. In real life, no transformer is 100% efficient at maintaining power output. However, for the BMAT questions will often assume that this is the case. Hence, when questions ask you about the power output of transformers, remember that:

$$\text{power output (W)}$$

$$= \text{voltage in primary coil (V)} \times \text{current in primary coil (A)}$$

$$= \text{voltage in secondary coil (V)} \times \text{current in secondary coil (A)}$$

> **Top Tip:** Note that current, power and velocity are all examples of *rates* – i.e. a description of how much a certain variable (charge, energy and displacement respectively in this case) changes per unit of time. Therefore, it is possible to express all rates as the *gradient* on a graph where the independent variable is time. The gradient can, of course, be worked out by dividing the change in the value on the y-axis by the change in time. In situations where you are asked to work out a rate from the gradient of a line on a graph, always make sure you use a section of the line that is completely straight! Otherwise your calculations may be wrong. Be warned – BMAT examiners may put in graphs that contain very subtle curves... Always check before starting your calculations.

1.7 Power generation

An electrical current will be generated whenever an electrical conductor is moved relative to a magnetic field *or* when a stationary conductor is exposed to a fluctuating magnetic field.

A **generator** may consist of a **wire coil** rotating in a **magnetic field**. As it rotates, each side of the coil moves through the magnetic field in *two different directions* with each turn. Because the wire is constantly 'switching' how it moves through the magnetic field as it rotates, an **alternating current** is generated.

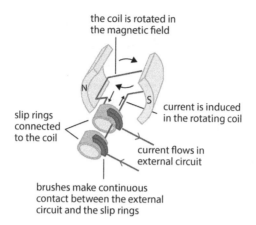

the coil is rotated in
the magnetic field

N

S

slip rings
connected
to the coil

current is induced
in the rotating coil

current flows in
external circuit

brushes make continuous
contact between the external
circuit and the slip rings

2. Motion and energy

2.1 Kinematics

You need to know that **speed** is a **scalar** quantity; when we know the speed of an object, we only know how fast it is travelling.

$$speed\ (m/s) = \frac{distance\ travelled\ (m)}{time\ (s)}$$

During a particular journey, an object may alter its speed several times. Hence we use the concept of **average speed** which is defined as **total distance travelled in a journey** divided by **total travel time**.

Velocity is a **vector** quantity. It describes how fast an object is travelling *in a certain direction*.

$$velocity\ (m/s) = \frac{distance\ travelled\ in\ a\ particular\ direction\ (m)}{time\ (s)}$$

Acceleration is also a **vector** quantity. It describes the rate of change in *velocity*. **Deceleration** is the same as acceleration, but with a negative value.

$$acceleration\ (m/s^2) = \frac{change\ in\ velocity\ (m/s)}{change\ in\ time\ (s)}$$

> **Top Tip:** Beware of the vector definitions of velocity and acceleration. It is possible for an object to have a *constant* speed but a *changing* velocity if the direction in which the object is moving is constantly changing. This may be true, for instance, in circular motion (a satellite orbiting, a car going around a bend). Of course, if the velocity of an object is changing the object is accelerating; and if the object is accelerating it follows that a net force is acting upon it. So keep in mind a car going around a bend at a constant speed is technically accelerating!

In a **distance–time** graph:

- A horizontal line will be recorded for a stationary object.
- A straight, diagonal line will be recorded for an object moving at a constant speed/velocity.
- Speed/velocity is equal to the gradient of the line. Lines with a steeper gradient represent a faster speed/velocity.
- The distance can be read directly off the *y*-axis.

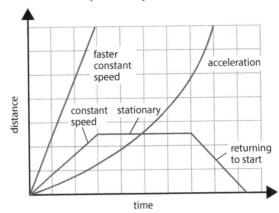

- A curved line will be recorded for an object that is accelerating.

In a **velocity–time** graph:

- A horizontal line will be recorded for an object with a constant speed/velocity.
- A straight, diagonal line will be recorded for an object with a constant acceleration.
- Acceleration is equal to the gradient of the line. Lines with steeper gradients represent greater accelerations.

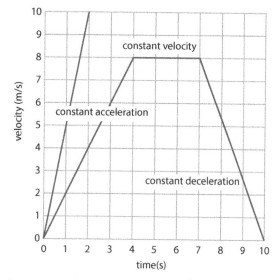

- The distance travelled is equal to the area under the graph.

2.2 Newton's Laws

Newton's First Law

An object will remain **stationary** or moving at a **constant velocity** unless acted on by an **unbalanced force**. Objects with **balanced** forces acting upon them will either be stationary or moving at a constant velocity (it may help to imagine a stationary object as having a velocity of 0 m/s!)

When an unbalanced force acts upon an object, the object will **accelerate** in the direction of that force.

Newton's Second Law

The acceleration of an object is *directly* proportional to the **net force** acting on the object and *inversely* proportional to the **mass** of the object. This is usually summarised with the equation:

$$net\ force\ (N) = mass\ (kg) \times acceleration\ (m/s^2)$$

Newton's Third Law

'For every action there is an equal and opposite reaction.' When two objects interact with each other, the force exerted on one object by the other will be equal, but opposite in direction, to the force exerted by the second object on the first object.

2.3 Momentum

An object's **momentum (p)** is defined as its **mass** multiplied by its **velocity**. It has units of **kilogram-metres per second**. Momentum is always *conserved* in a system. That means that if a moving object collides with a stationary object, the *total* momentum of both objects after the collision will be equal to the momentum of the moving object before the collision.

For any change in momentum to occur, a force must be applied. The size of a force that acts on an object to alter its momentum is equal to the rate of change in that momentum, or:

$$\text{force (N)} = \frac{\text{change in momentum (kg m/s)}}{\text{change in time (s)}}$$

Cars include safety features such as **seatbelts** and **crumple zones**. In the event of a collision, these safety features slow down the deceleration of passengers inside the vehicle. Consequently, the change in the passengers' momentum occurs over a longer period of time and they are exposed to smaller forces. This reduces the possibility of injury.

> **Top Tip:** Momentum questions can often involve guns or cannons – remember that the momentum of the stationary gun (i.e. 0 kgm/s) is equal to the combined momentums of the fired projectile and the recoiling gun. This is because the two objects move in opposite directions, so if we assign the projectile a positive velocity, the gun will have a negative velocity.

2.4 Mass, weight and free-fall

Mass is defined as the quantity of matter in an object. It is measured in **kilograms (kg)**.

Weight is defined as the *force acting on an object* due to the effects of **gravity**. It is measured, like any other force, in **newtons (N)**.

The weight of an object is calculated as its **mass** multiplied by the **acceleration due to gravity** (*g*). For the purposes of the BMAT, you should assume $g = 10$ m/s^2.

When an object is in **free-fall**, it has two forces acting on it that determine how fast it falls – its **weight** and its **aerodynamic drag**. Free-fall has several stages:

- Initially, the weight of the object is greater than drag, causing the object to accelerate.
- As the object gets faster, drag increases.
- Drag increases until the point when it is *equal* to weight.
- At this point, forces acting upon the object are balanced and the object falls at a constant speed. This is known as **terminal velocity**.

Skydivers will fall for a certain time at a *fast* terminal velocity. They will then deploy their parachute, which causes the drag force to increase dramatically. This results in deceleration (as drag is greater than weight). However, as the parachutist slows down, drag decreases. The parachutist decelerates until they reach a new, slower terminal velocity. Note that at the new terminal velocity, the values of weight and drag will still be the same as their values at the *previous* terminal velocity.

> **Top Tip:** Remember that a skydiver falling at terminal velocity will have a drag force acting upon them that is equal to their weight, no matter the speed at which they fall.

2.5 Energy

Energy is defined as the capacity to do work. **Work done** is equal to energy transferred. Energy and work are both measured in **joules (J)**.

$$work\ done\ (J) = force\ (N) \times distance\ (m)$$

Note that the distance over which a force is applied *must* be in the same direction in which the force is acting for the equation to work. For example, if we move an object of a certain weight *horizontally* for a certain distance, we cannot work out the work done by multiplying the weight by the distance travelled. This is because weight is a *vertically acting* force.

Instead, the relevant force to use in the equation is the *driving force* that moves the object horizontally.

As mentioned above, **power (P)** is the rate of energy transfer:

$$power\ (W) = \frac{energy\ (J)}{time\ (s)}$$

Gravitational potential energy, or just **potential energy (PE)**, is the energy gained by an object as it is moved to a higher position.

$$change\ in\ potential\ energy\ (J)$$
$$= mass\ (kg) \times acceleration\ due\ to\ gravity\ (m/s^2) \times change\ in\ height\ (m)$$

An object's **kinetic energy** is the energy possessed by a moving object.

$$kinetic\ energy\ (J) = \tfrac{1}{2} \times mass\ (kg) \times (velocity\ (m/s))^2$$

Top Tip: If an object falls, all of its potential energy *must* be converted into a different type of energy. In cases where there is no drag, or drag is negligible, *all* the potential energy must be converted into kinetic energy. But be careful: if there is drag, some of the potential energy will be converted into energy of other types, e.g. heat and sound. Note the opposite is also true – whenever an object is lifted, some energy *must* be expended to be converted into potential energy.

Energy is always **conserved**; it is not created or destroyed, but converted from one type to another. The different types of energy are:

- Heat
- Light
- Sound
- Kinetic
- Electric
- Nuclear
- Elastic potential
- Gravitational potential
- Chemical potential

Often we want to convert energy from one type into another type that is *useful* to us; i.e. it allows us to do *useful* work. However, no energy conversion is perfectly efficient, and there will always be some energy 'lost' in forms that are *not* useful to us. Often energy losses are in the form of heat.

$$energy\ efficiency\ (\%) = \frac{useful\ energy\ output\ (J)}{total\ energy\ output\ (J)} \times 100\%$$

3. Thermal physics and matter

3.1 Matter

Matter is made up of many small **particles** (e.g. molecules, atoms, ions, etc.) These particles behave differently in different **phases** of matter.

In **solids**, particles are tightly packed together and are only able to vibrate around a fixed point. As they are heated, these particles will vibrate more and gain more energy until they are able to overcome, to an extent, the bonds holding them close together. At this point, **melting** occurs, and the solid will change into a liquid.

In **liquids**, particles are not fixed in their position and they are free to move around each other. However, they are limited in how far they can move away from each other. As particles gain more energy by heating, they are able to overcome the bonds that keep them associated with their neighbours.

As a liquid is heated, particles may gain enough energy to **evaporate**. This is defined as the transition of particles from a liquid to gas phase at the *surface* of the liquid. As the temperature increases, the rate of evaporation increases.

If the temperature of the substance reaches a sufficient level, particles may escape from the bonds to their neighbours at *any location* within the body of liquid (i.e. not just at the surface). When gas is formed throughout the liquid and not just at the surface, we say the liquid is **boiling**.

In a **gas**, particles are free to move independently of other particles. Hence, particles in a gas may have relatively large spaces between them.

As heat is applied to matter, the average volume occupied by any particle increases. This means that as substances are heated, they become less dense. **Density (ρ – rho)** is defined as:

$$density\ (kg/m^3) = \frac{mass\ (kg)}{volume\ (m^3)}$$

3.2 Transfer of heat

Heat energy will always move from regions of high temperature to regions of a lower temperature. Heat energy is also called internal energy, because the heat of a substance is determined by the kinetic energy of the particles within that substance. Heat transfer, or the transfer of kinetic energy between particles, occurs through three different routes, as follows.

Conduction

Conduction is the transfer of energy through **solids**. Within solids, particles are packed tightly together and they are immobile, apart from vibrating in a fixed position. As they gain more energy, they vibrate more. In doing so, they collide with neighbouring particles and pass on some of their energy. The vibration of particles is the basis of heat energy.

Thermal **insulators** do not conduct heat well. This may be because their particles are less densely packed, which makes collision events less likely to occur, or because they contain pockets of air (air is a poor conductor because its particles are spread out).

Thermal **conductors** conduct heat well. Metal is a good thermal conductor because it contains **free electrons**. These electrons can move independently of the metal cations; they can also gain kinetic energy as the metal is heated. When high-kinetic energy electrons collide with other particles, they pass on some of their energy.

Conduction is a relatively quick transfer of heat energy, because collisions between vibrating particles and their neighbours are very likely to occur.

Convection

Convection is the transfer of heat through **fluids**. Particles within fluids (liquids and gases) are not as densely packed as in solids, hence they are less likely to collide. Instead, as fluid particles gain more kinetic energy, they occupy a greater **volume** of space. Therefore, a hot region of fluid will be *less dense* than a cooler region of fluid. As a result, the hot fluid rises above the cool fluid, and the cool fluid takes the place of the hot fluid next to the source of heat. A **convection current** is established as different regions of fluid fluctuate in density. Gradually, the convection current spreads heat throughout the body of fluid.

The effectiveness of convection currents at transferring heat can be affected by properties of the fluid itself, such as viscosity.

Radiation

Heat can also be transferred as radiation; specifically, as **infrared (IR) radiation**. IR radiation is a type of **electromagnetic radiation**, and it exists in the form of waves of energy (or photons).

All objects absorb and emit IR radiation. The hotter an object, the more IR radiation it emits.

Objects with a **large surface area** will emit more IR radiation than an object of identical mass and temperature, but with a smaller surface area.

Dark, matt surfaces are better at emitting *and* absorbing IR radiation than **shiny or reflective surfaces**.

4. Waves

4.1 Wave nature

A **wave** is a transfer of energy through matter which results in no *net* displacement of particles of that matter. Energy instead is transferred by particles oscillating around a fixed point.

Electromagnetic waves are slightly different, insomuch as they consist of oscillations within electrical and magnetic fields (see below).

Transverse waves are ones in which the direction of travel and energy transfer is *perpendicular* to the direction of the oscillation of the particles. Water waves and seismic 'S' waves are transverse waves.

Longitudinal waves are ones in which the direction of travel and energy transfer is *parallel* to the direction of the oscillation of the particles. Sound waves and seismic 'P' waves are longitudinal waves.

In waves:

- The **amplitude** is the *maximum* distance that a particle moves from an undisturbed position.
- The **frequency** (*f*) is the number of cycles of a wave that pass a fixed point in one second. It is measured in **hertz (Hz)** or 'per second' (s^{-1}). Waves with a higher frequency have a lower wavelength.

- The **time period** is the time taken for a single cycle to fully pass a fixed point.
- The **wavelength (λ)** is the distance between one point on a wave and the equivalent point on the following wave. Waves with a greater wavelength have a lower frequency.

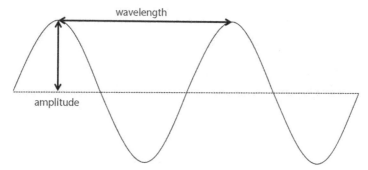

- The **wave-speed** is how quickly the wave travels.

These concepts are linked by a couple of equations:

$$wave\text{-}speed~(m/s) = frequency~(Hz) \times wavelength~(m)$$

$$time~period~(s) = \frac{1}{frequency~(Hz)}$$

4.2 Wave behaviour

All waves can be **reflected**. Remember that the angle of **incidence is equal** to the **angle of reflection**. Note that these angles are between the wave and the normal (i.e. the line perpendicular to the boundary between the two media).

When a wave reaches a boundary between two different substances of different densities, it may be **refracted** – this is simply a change in direction. As a wave enters a *denser* medium, its direction of travel is shifted *closer* to the normal.

If a wave crosses a boundary at 90°, it will not be refracted.

If a wave moving from a *dense* medium to a *less dense* medium hits the boundary at an angle known as the **critical angle**, the wave will be refracted along the boundary.

If it hits the boundary at an angle *greater than* the critical angle, it will reflect back into the denser medium. This is known as **total internal reflection**.

4.3 The Doppler effect

If a wave source moves *towards* an object, the receiver encounters waves that are *higher in frequency* than the frequency at which the source produces the waves. This is because waves will 'bunch up' in front of the moving wave source.

Conversely, if the wave source moves *away* from an object, the receiver is exposed to waves that are *lower in frequency* than the frequency at which the source produces waves. This is because waves will 'spread out' behind the moving object.

This is known as the **Doppler effect**.

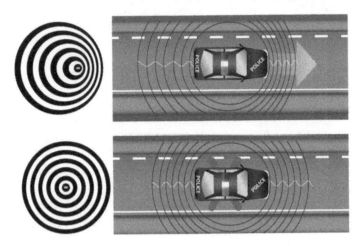

4.4 Sound waves

Sound waves are longitudinal waves that are transmitted through matter.

When a sound wave is reflected, this is called an **echo**.

Ultrasound describes any sound wave that is above the frequency threshold of human hearing. It can be used for:

- **Imaging** human tissues; at boundaries between different tissues, some ultrasound is reflected. By calculating the time taken between emitting an ultrasound wave and receiving its echo, computers can build up an image of the interior of the body.
- **Echolocation** in animals; bats produce ultrasound waves. By calculating the time taken between emitting an ultrasound wave and receiving its echo, they can determine the location of their prey.

4.5 Electromagnetic waves

Electromagnetic (EM) waves are transverse waves made from fluctuations in magnetic and electric fields. *All* EM waves travel at the speed of light; in a vacuum the speed of light is approximately 300,000 km/s.

EM waves of different *frequencies* fall into different categories. The different types of EM wave that exist make up the **EM radiation spectrum**. Each different type of radiation has its own practical uses and associated dangers. They are listed in the table below in order of increasing frequency:

Name of wave	Frequency	Wavelength	Uses	Dangers
Radio	Lowest	Longest	• Communications • **Low-frequency** radio waves can be *diffracted* around large obstacles like hills, so transmitters do not necessarily need to be in sight of the receiver. • **High-frequency** radio waves can be reflected off the **ionosphere**, a charged region of the atmosphere; this allows them to be sent around the Earth.	None
Microwave			• **Cooking**: microwaves can be absorbed by water molecules in food, causing the food to heat up. • **Communications**: mobile phone signals are transmitted as microwaves. Microwaves will also pass directly through the Earth's atmosphere, and can be used for satellite communication.	Can heat tissues and cause burns
Infrared			• Used in electric heaters, toasters, grills. • Also used in fibre-optic cables; total internal reflection of IR radiation along a cable is used to transmit messages.	Can cause burns
Visible light*			• Used to see. • Used in **lasers**.	High intensities of light can damage eyes
Ultraviolet			• Used in sunbeds. • Objects that **fluoresce** (e.g. fluorescent lights, security markings on bank notes) absorb UV light and re-emit it as visible light.	Can cause sunburn and skin cancer
X-ray			• Used for **medical imaging**, as it passes through soft tissue, but is not transmitted by dense tissues such as bone. • Used to detect metal objects and welds for cracks.	Can cause cancer. As ionising radiation, can also cause radiation sickness

Name of wave	Frequency	Wavelength	Uses	Dangers
Gamma	Highest	Shortest	• **Sterilisation** of medical equipment. • **Cancer radiotherapy** – exposing a tumour to gamma rays from several different angles helps to kill the cancer while limiting damage to surrounding tissue.	Can cause cancer. As ionising radiation, can also cause radiation sickness.

Note that the lowest frequency visible light is red light and the highest frequency visible light is violet light.

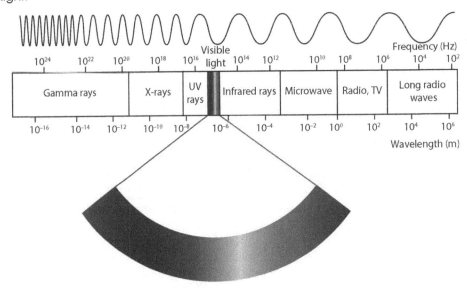

5. Radioactivity

5.1 Types of decay

The atoms of some elements have unstable nuclei. This may be because the nucleus is too *large*, because the number of protons is very different to the number of neutrons or because the nucleus has a lot of energy. In order to become more stable, nuclei will emit **radiation**.

There are three types of radioactive decay: alpha, beta and gamma. They each have different characteristics. All three types of decay produce **ionising radiation**; i.e. radiation that can free electrons from atoms and produce ions.

Alpha decay

Alpha decay occurs when an **alpha particle** is ejected from the nucleus. An alpha particle is made up of **two neutrons** and **two protons**. Hence it is equivalent to a **helium nucleus**. Alpha particles are *highly ionising* because of their relative large size. However, they are also relatively slow-moving and *weakly penetrating*: they can be stopped by a **few centimetres of air**.

When an alpha particle is ejected from the nucleus of an atom, the atom is **transmuted** into a different element. This is because it has *lost* two protons, and so its **atomic number** drops by two. In addition, because of the loss of the two neutrons, its **atomic mass** drops by *four*. Here is an example of radon–219 decaying into polonium–215:

$$^{219}_{86}\text{Rn} \rightarrow {}^{215}_{84}\text{Po} + {}^{4}_{2}\text{He}^{2+}$$

Top Tip: Don't confuse an alpha particle with a helium *atom* – the latter also has two electrons.

Beta decay

Beta decay occurs when a **beta particle** is ejected from the nucleus. A beta particle is an **electron**. In the nucleus, a neutron turns into a proton and an electron (which is ejected). Hence the atom is transmuted to an element with an atomic number that is *greater by one*. For this reason we also say that beta particles have an atomic number of '-1'. The mass of the nucleus remains unchanged as the total number of protons and neutrons will remain the same. Here is an example of carbon–14 decaying into nitrogen–14:

$$^{14}_{6}\text{C} \rightarrow {}^{14}_{7}\text{N} + {}^{0}_{-1}\text{e}^{-}$$

Top Tip: The electron released during beta decay comes from the nucleus, not the electron shell. If the electron were to be released from the electron shell, it would create an ion instead.

It is also possible for the beta particle that is produced to be a **positron** – the positively charged antimatter counterpart of an electron. When a *positron* is lost, a **proton** changes into a **neutron** and atomic number *decreases* by one. Here is an example of magnesium–23 decaying into sodium–23:

$$^{23}_{12}\text{Mg} \rightarrow {}^{23}_{11}\text{Na} + \text{e}^{+}$$

Beta particles are *moderately ionising, moderately fast-moving* and *moderately penetrating*; they can be stopped by **aluminium foil**.

Gamma decay

Gamma decay occurs when **gamma radiation** is emitted from the nucleus (i.e. a high-energy **photon**). The atom does not change in mass or atomic number.

Gamma radiation is relatively *weakly ionising*, but it is *highly penetrating*. It can only be stopped by **thick lead**.

> **Top Tip:** Examiners may use radioactive decay in order to combine concepts from physics and chemistry. Remember, if an atom decays and changes element, its electronic configuration and reactivity will change too.

5.2 Uses and dangers of different radioactivity

Alpha particles are used in **smoke alarms**. An alpha source in the alarm emits particles that ionise air molecules. The ions that are produced carry a current and complete a circuit within the alarm. Smoke particles prevent the ionisation of air molecules from occurring – this reduces the current. When this happens, the alarm sounds.

Because alpha particles are so highly ionising, they are extremely dangerous to cells and tissues because they can damage DNA. However, because they are so weakly penetrating they only present a danger when **ingested** or **inhaled**.

Beta particles are used to examine the thickness of materials such as paper and aluminium sheets as they are produced in factories. If the material gets too thick, fewer particles will penetrate through it. This can be detected using a radiation detector.

In addition, certain **tracers** can be made that produce beta particles. In medicine, a chemical that accumulates in a certain part of the body can be artificially made to release beta particles. Recording the production of these beta particles using techniques such as **positron emission topography (PET)** can allow us to image the relevant area of the body.

Beta particles are moderately penetrating, and so they represent a danger if they are inhaled or ingested *or* if a person is exposed to them directly without a barrier to protect them.

Gamma radiation is used to sterilise medical equipment and food. It is also used in cancer radiotherapy, where a tumour is exposed to gamma rays from several different directions.

As gamma rays are weakly ionising, they do not present a significant danger when given in very small doses. In radiotherapy, changing the direction from which the tumour is exposed to gamma rays minimises exposure in surrounding healthy tissue. However, gamma rays are highly penetrating, and thus present a danger in high doses (since only a thick lead or concrete barrier will prevent exposure).

All types of ionising radiation can cause radiation burns, radiation sickness and cancer.

5.3 Half-life

Radioactive decay is a completely random process – we can have an idea of the **probability** that a certain nucleus will decay in a given period, but we cannot *definitely* say when it will decay.

The **half-life** of a radioactive substance is the time taken for 50% of the atoms in the substance to decay, or the time taken for the **count-rate** of a substance to decrease by 50%. The radioactive count can be measured using a Geiger counter and is measured in Becquerels (Bq), where 1 Bq is one nucleus decay per second.

The half-life for any given radioactive isotope is *constant*. It cannot be altered, for instance, by changing external factors such as temperature and pressure.

> **Top Tip:** Remember that there will always be a base level of radioactive count rate due to background radiation, caused by cosmic rays, radon gas, radioactive rocks, etc.

5.4 Nuclear fission

The breaking apart of a nucleus is known as **nuclear fission**. Nuclear fission releases a lot of energy that is stored within the nucleus. Currently, nuclear fission is the basis of providing energy in nuclear power plants.

You need to know specifically about the fission of uranium-235. In the fission reaction, a nucleus of uranium-235 absorbs a neutron. This produces uranium-236, which is unstable. The uranium-236 fissures into two smaller nuclei, which are radioactive, releasing three neutrons in the process. Here is the equation of the fission of uranium-235 to produce krypton and barium (note that krypton and barium are not the *only* possible products; other elements may be produced too):

$$^{235}_{92}U + ^{1}_{0}n \rightarrow ^{90}_{36}Kr + ^{143}_{56}Ba + ^{1}_{0}n + ^{1}_{0}n + ^{1}_{0}n$$

The three neutrons may then be absorbed by three other uranium-235 nuclei and the process continues. This is known as a **chain reaction**. In power plants, some of the neutrons are 'soaked up' using carbon rods to control the chain reaction. An uncontrolled chain reaction can lead to a **nuclear explosion**.

5.5 Nuclear fusion

When two atomic nuclei are fused together, this is **nuclear fusion**. This is the source of energy produced by the sun. Fusion requires *extremely* high temperatures to occur, as the nuclei need to have enough energy to overcome their mutual charge repulsion.

In the sun, fusion occurs predominantly between hydrogen nuclei to form helium. The reaction requires two different isotopes of hydrogen: hydrogen-1 and hydrogen-2 (also known as deuterium).

$$^{1}_{1}H + ^{2}_{1}H \rightarrow ^{3}_{2}He$$

Maths

1. Number

For the exam, you need to be comfortable performing addition, subtraction, division and multiplication *without* a calculator – see the section on how to do maths without a calculator (p. 108).

1.1 Multiples and factors

A **multiple** of a number, x, can be divided by x and not leave a remainder.

A **factor** of a number, x, is one that x will divide by without leaving a remainder.

The **highest common factor (HCF)** is the highest factor that is shared between two numbers.

The **lowest common multiple (LCM)** is the lowest multiple that is shared between two numbers.

A **prime number** is a number *greater than 1* that only has factors of itself and 1.

Prime factorisation can be used to establish the HCF and LCM of two or more numbers. The highest common factor will simply be the combination of prime factors that is shared between all numbers, and the lowest common multiple will be the prime factors of both numbers multiplied together, but removing any sets of numbers that are repeated:

$$1092 = 2 \times 2 \times 3 \times 7 \times 13$$

$$588 = 2 \times 2 \times 3 \times 7 \times 7$$

$$HCF = 2 \times 2 \times 3 \times 7 = 84$$

$$LCM = 2 \times 2 \times 3 \times 7 \times 7 \times 13 = 7644$$

1.2 Index laws

A number to the power of n is that number multiplied by itself n times:

$$2^4 = 2 \times 2 \times 2 \times 2 = 16$$

A number to the power of $-n$ is equal to 1 divided by that number to the power of n:

$$2^{-4} = \frac{1}{2^4} = \frac{1}{2 \times 2 \times 2 \times 2} = \frac{1}{16}$$

A number to the power of $\frac{1}{n}$ is equal to the nth root of that number:

$$2^{\frac{1}{4}} = \sqrt[4]{2} = 1.1892\ldots$$

Note also the following index laws:

$$x^a\, x^b = x^{a+b}$$

$$x^a/x^b = x^{a-b}$$

$$(x^a)^b = x^{ab}$$

1.3 Standard Index Form

Standard Index Form is a way of writing a number in the format $A \times 10^n$.

A is always a number between 1 and 10.

n tells us where the decimal point lies – if n is positive, we move the decimal point n places to the *right*. If n is negative, we move the decimal point n places to the *left*.

$$5.2 \times 10^6 = 5,200,000$$

$$3.7 \times 10^{-4} = 0.00037$$

To multiply standard form numbers, multiply the A values separately and then *add* the n values:

$$3 \times 10^4 \times 4 \times 10^3 = 12 \times 10^7 = 1.2 \times 10^8$$

To divide standard form numbers divide the A values separately and then *subtract* the n values:

$$(4 \times 10^5) \div (2 \times 10^3) = 2 \times 10^2$$

1.4 Fraction, decimal and percentage

You need to be comfortable converting between fractions, decimals and percentages without a calculator. Below is a table of conversions of common fractions that you may find useful:

Fraction	Decimal	Per cent	Fraction	Decimal	Per cent
1/2	0.5	50%	1/8	0.125	12.5%
1/3	0.333...	33.333...%	3/8	0.375	37.5%
2/3	0.666...	66.666...%	5/8	0.625	62.5%
1/4	0.25	25%	7/8	0.875	87.5%
3/4	0.75	75%	1/9	0.111...	11.111...%
1/5	0.2	20%	2/9	0.222...	22.222...%
2/5	0.4	40%	4/9	0.444...	44.444...%
3/5	0.6	60%	5/9	0.555...	55.555...%
4/5	0.8	80%	7/9	0.777...	77.777...%
1/6	0.1666...	16.666...%	8/9	0.888...	88.888...%
5/6	0.8333...	83.333...%	1/10	0.1	10%
			1/12	0.08333...	8.333...%
			1/16	0.0625	6.25%
			1/32	0.03125	3.125%

Top Tip: 1/7 and its multiples demonstrate an interesting characteristic: when expressed as decimals or percentages, the repeated sequence of numbers '142857' will always appear.
1/7 = 0.1428571428...
2/7 = 0.2857142857...
3/7 = 0.4285714285...

1.5 Percentages and percentage change

To work out X% of a number, divide X by 100 and then multiply it by that number.

$$50\% \text{ of } 76 = (50 \div 100) \times 76 = 0.5 \times 76 = 38$$

When a number is *increased* by X%, multiply that number by $1 + (X \div 100)$.

$$\text{Increase 76 by } 50\% = (1 + 0.5) \times 76 = 1.5 \times 76 = 114$$

When a number is *decreased* by $X\%$, multiply that number by $1 - (X \div 100)$.

$$\text{Decrease 76 by 25\%} = (1 - 0.25) \times 76 = 0.75 \times 76 = 57$$

1.6 Ratios

A **ratio** is simply another way of writing a fraction. Like fractions, they can be simplified:

$$12{:}15 = 3{:}5$$

If, in a class, the ratio of boys to girls is 12:15, boys make up 12/27 of the class and girls make up 15/27 – the denominator of the fraction can be found by the total of the numbers in the ratio.

1.7 Proportion

When two numbers are **directly proportional**, if one number increases the other number increases *by the same factor*. If two numbers a and b are directly proportional:

$$a \propto b$$

$$a = kb, \text{ where } k \text{ is a constant}$$

Knowing a given value of a and b allows you to work out k, which means that you can then work out all values of b for any value of a and vice versa.

When two numbers are **inversely proportional**, if one number increases the other number *decreases by the same factor*. If two numbers a and b are inversely proportional:

$$a \propto 1/b$$

$$a = k/b$$

Again, k is a constant that can be worked out to establish all values of a and b.

1.8 Surds

A surd is a square root that cannot be converted to a rational number. There are some rules that can be used to simplify surds:

$$\sqrt{a} \times \sqrt{b} = \sqrt{ab}$$

$$\sqrt{a} \times \sqrt{a} = a$$

$$\frac{\sqrt{a}}{\sqrt{b}} = \sqrt{\frac{a}{b}}$$

You may be asked to rationalise the denominator of a fraction containing a surd. To do this, multiply that fraction by the surd divided by itself (= 1).

$$\frac{x}{\sqrt{a}} = \frac{x}{\sqrt{a}} \times \frac{\sqrt{a}}{\sqrt{a}} = \frac{x\sqrt{a}}{a}$$

1.9 Approximations

When a number is rounded to a certain number of **significant figures**, you include the stated number of digits *starting from the first non-zero digit*.

0.032012 to 4 s.f. is 0.03201

When a number is rounded to a certain number of **decimal places**, you include the stated number of digits *starting from the digit after the decimal point*.

0.032012 to 4 d.p. is 0.0320

When rounding, if the proceeding digit is *less than* 5, you round down. If the proceeding digit is *5 or greater* you round up.

If we are told a value that has been rounded, the **upper bound** or **maximum** of that value is the limit at which we would *round up*.

So if I have a plank of wood that is 14 cm long to 2 s.f., its **upper bound** must be 14.5 cm. At that value and above I would round *up* to 15 cm.

Similarly, the **lower bound** or **minimum** of that value is the limit at which we would *round down*.

So the **lower bound** of the plank's length is 13.5 cm. Below this value we would round *down* to a length of 13 cm.

2. Algebra

2.1 Algebraic operations

You need to be comfortable with the following concepts:

- Multiplying out of a bracket:

$$a(b + c) = ab + ac$$

- Expanding the product of two linear expressions:

$$(a + b)(c + d) = ac + ad + bc + bd$$

- Factorising:

$$ab + ac = a(b + c)$$

You need to be able to simplify rational expressions by cancelling.

To do this, you have to be able to recognise common factors that are present in both the numerator and the denominator of a fraction. This may only become possible when certain expressions are factorised.

$$\frac{a^2 + ab}{ab} = \frac{a(a + b)}{ab} = \frac{a + b}{b}$$

2.2 Simultaneous equations

To solve simultaneous equations in two unknowns, you should have enough information to describe one of the unknowns in terms of the other. From here, you can solve a simple linear equation:

$$2a + b = 3$$

$$3a + 2b = 5$$

$$b = 3 - 2a$$

$$3a + 2(3 - 2a) = 3a + 6 - 4a = 6 - a = 5$$

$$a = 1$$

$$b = 1$$

2.3 Quadratic equations

You need to be able to solve quadratic equations. In order to do this, the expression needs to first be factorised.

A quadratic equation will be in the form $ax^2 + bx + c = 0$

The factorised equation will be in the form $(mx + n)(px + q) = 0$

You need to find values for m, n, p and q that satisfy these criteria:

$$mp = a$$

$$nq = c$$

$$np + mq = b$$

Hence the equation $2x^2 + 8x + 6 = 0$ factorises to $(2x + 2)(x + 3) = 0$

Then solve each factor as an independent equation:

$$x + 3 = 0$$

$$x = -3$$

$$2x + 2 = 0$$

$$2x = -2$$

$$x = -1$$

$$x = -1 \text{ and } -3$$

> **Top Tip:** Remember two quick methods for helping to solve quadratic equations:
>
> - Completing the square:
>
> $x^2 + 10x + 21 = (x + 5)^2 - 4$; note: this is a useful method for solving expressions that do not factorise easily.
>
> - Finding the difference of two squares:
>
> $x^2 - 25 = (x + 5)(x - 5)$; 25 can be replaced with any square number.

2.4 Inequalities

For the BMAT, you only need to learn how to solve *linear* inequalities.

Usually, solving inequalities can be carried out in much the same way that you would solve a simple, linear algebraic equation:

$$3x + 3 > 5$$

$$3x > 2$$

$$x > 2/3$$

However, remember that if you're *dividing* or *multiplying* by a negative number on both sides of the equation, the direction of the inequality *switches*:

$$-3x + 3 > 5$$

$$-3x > 2$$

$$x < -2/3$$

2.5 Sequences

To solve arithmetic sequences:

- Identify the difference between the terms in the sequence.
- Identify the *number* of the term in the sequence. For instance, if you had the third term in the sequence, you would have term number 3.
- Find the difference between the term number and the term itself.

So if our sequence was 2, 5, 8, 11…

The difference between the terms is 3.

Term number 1 is '2'. The difference between 1 and 2 is $1 - 2 = -1$

So our expression for the *n*th term is $3n - 1$

You may have to express a **quadratic sequence**. This occurs when the differences between terms are different, but there is a constant difference between differences. For example:

1, 3, 7, 13, 21, 31

The differences are 2, 4, 6, 8, 10.

The differences between the differences is always 2.

For these sequences, the expression describing the *n*th term always contains n^2.

If the difference between the differences is x, then the n^2 part of the expression is given by $x/2(n^2)$.

Hence, if the difference of the differences is 2, then the expression uses n^2.

If the difference of the differences is 3, the expression uses $1.5n^2$.

If the difference of the differences is 4, the expression uses $2n^2$.

If it is 6, we use $3n^2$, and so on.

For the above sequence, where the difference between the differences is 2, the n^2 part of the expression is just n^2.

In the next step, subtract the n^2 parts from the corresponding terms in the sequence; this should leave a simple arithmetic sequence.

Hence:

Sequence: 1, 3, 7, 13, 21, 31

n^2 part: 1, 4, 9, 16, 25, 36

Difference: 0, –1, –2, –3, –4, –5

Then work out the expression of the arithmetic sequence that is produced.

Here it is: $-n + 1$.

Then combine this arithmetic sequence expression with your n^2 term to get the expression for your quadratic sequence.

Hence, our quadratic sequence expression in this case is $n^2 - n + 1$.

2.6 Graphs

You should recognise that straight line graphs are usually written in the form $y = mx + c$ where m is the gradient of the line and c is the y-intercept.

You need to be able to graphically solve linear equations where one equation is quadratic and one is linear. To do this, simply read off where the lines intercept.

You should be able to recognise the following graphs in all 4 Cartesian quadrants:

Quadratic functions – e.g. $y = x^2$

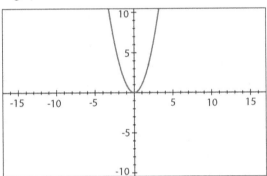

Cubic functions – e.g. $y = x^3$

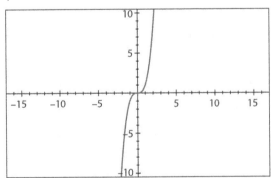

Reciprocal functions – e.g. y = 1/x

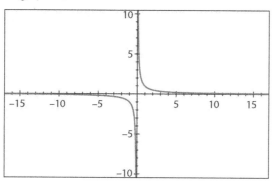

y = sin x

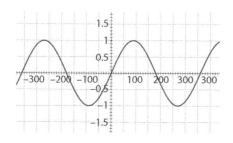

y = cos x

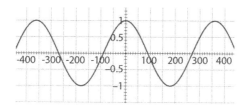

y = tan x

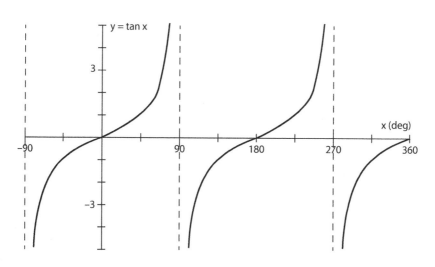

Exponential functions – e.g. $y = 2^x$

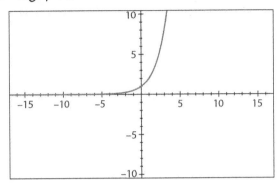

You also need to be able to recognise the following transformations of functions:

Let $y = f(x)$ be a function of a graph –

$y = af(x)$ is a stretch by a factor of a along the y-axis.

$y = f(ax)$ is a stretch by a factor of $\dfrac{1}{a}$ along the x-axis.

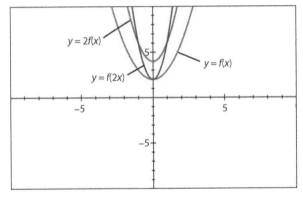

$y = f(x) + a$ is a translation of the line a units along the y-axis (in a *positive* direction).

$y = f(x + a)$ is a translation of the line a units along the x-axis (in a *negative* direction).

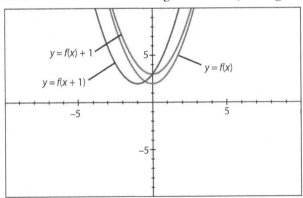

$y = -f(x)$ is a reflection of the line in the x-axis.

$y = f(-x)$ is a reflection of the line in the y-axis.

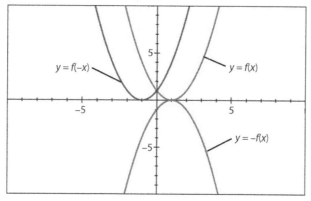

3. Geometry

3.1 Angles

Angles at a point add up to 360°.

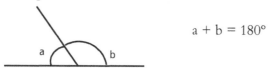

$$a + b + c + d = 360°$$

Angles on a straight line add up to 180°.

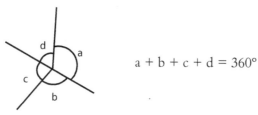

$$a + b = 180°$$

Opposite angles at a vertex are always equal.

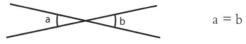

$$a = b$$

Parallel lines:

- Opposite angles are equal, $a = c$.
- Corresponding angles are equal, $a = b$.
- Alternate angles are equal, $b = c$.
- Co-interior angles add up to 180°, $c + d = 180°$.

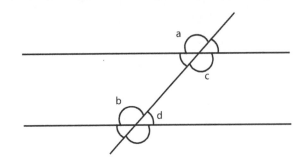

Interior angles in a triangle add up to 180°.

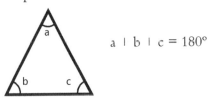

$a + b + c = 180°$

Interior angles in a quadrilateral add up to 360°.

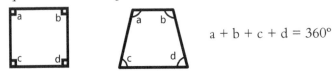

$a + b + c + d = 360°$

The exterior angles of any polygon always add up to 360°. Therefore, for any regular polygon of n sides, each exterior angle is equal to $360°/n$.

The interior angles of a regular polygon of n sides will each be equal to $(n − 2) × 180°$.

3.2 Congruence and similarity

Shapes are **congruent** if their sides are all the same length and they have the same corresponding angles.

Shapes are **similar** if one shape is congruent to an enlargement of the other.

Note that for similar shapes, if the length of a side of one shape is x times greater than the corresponding length on the other shape, the area will be x^2 times greater and the volume will be x^3 times greater.

For instance, say there are two similar cubes, A and B. Cube A has a side that is twice as large as the side of Cube B. This means that the area of a face of Cube A is four times greater than the area of a face of Cube B. The volume of Cube A is eight times larger than that of Cube B.

3.3 Triangles

You need to be familiar with Pythagoras' Theorem:

For a right-angled triangle with sides of length a, b and c, and where the side of length c is the hypotenuse:

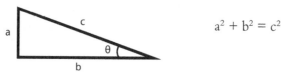

$$a^2 + b^2 = c^2$$

In a right-angled triangle with angle θ, the following relationships are true:

$$\frac{opposite}{hypotenuse} = \sin\theta$$

$$\frac{adjacent}{hypotenuse} = \cos\theta$$

$$\frac{opposite}{adjacent} = \frac{\sin\theta}{\cos\theta} = \tan\theta$$

For the BMAT, you just need to be aware of these relationships. You will *not* be expected to recall trigonometric values!

Top Tip: Often BMAT geometry questions will ask you to solve angles in 3D shapes; in addition, you probably won't have the angle 'drawn on' the diagram you're given. Instead, you will have to identify it yourself. For instance, you might be asked to 'find the sine of the angle ED makes with the horizontal plane' in the diagram below:

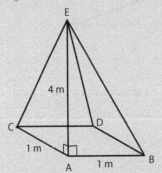

Don't be panicked by the wording! Simply identify the line ED and the *smallest* angle it could possibly make with a horizontal surface. Then work out sine (opposite divided by adjacent).

With questions asking you to solve the angle in a 3D shape, it's always best to work out the answer by splitting the shape up into several 2D shapes. Hence, for the question above, we *first* need to work out length AD using Pythagoras' Theorem:

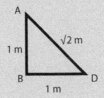

Then, to find the answer we need to find the sine of angle ADE. This is $4/\sqrt{2}$, or $2\sqrt{2}$:

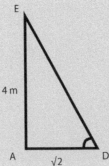

3.4 Circle theorems

Learn the following circle theorems:

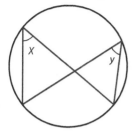

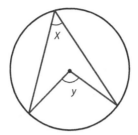

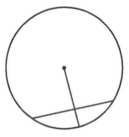

$x = y$, angles subtended by the same chord are equal

$y = 2x$, angles at the centre are double angles at the circumference subtended by the same chord

$x = 90°$, angles at the circumference subtended by the diameter are always equal to 90°

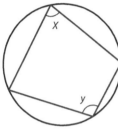

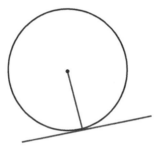

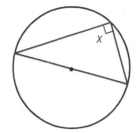

$x + y = 180°$, opposite angles in cyclic quadrilaterals add up to 180°

The radius is perpendicular to the tangent

The radius bisects a chord and is perpendicular to a chord

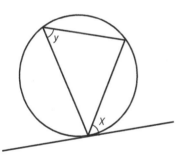

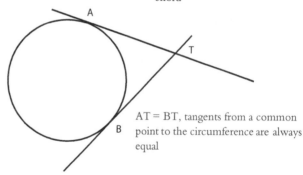

The angle between the tangent and chord at the point of contact is equal to the angle in the **alternate segment**

AT = BT, tangents from a common point to the circumference are always equal

4. Measures

4.1 Areas and perimeters

2D shapes

Shape	Area	Perimeter
Square	A² – where A is length of one side	4A
Rectangle	A × B – where A and B are lengths of perpendicular sides	2A + 2B
Triangle	½ × *base* × *height*	A + B + C – where A, B and C are lengths of sides
Parallelogram	*base* × *height*	2A + 2B – where A and B are non-parallel sides
Trapezium	((A + B)/2) × *height* – where A and B are lengths of parallel sides	A + B + C + D – total of all four sides

The **circumference** of a circle is given by $2\pi r$, where r is the radius.

The **area** of a circle is πr^2.

The **length of an arc** is given by $2\pi r\dfrac{x}{360}$, where x is the angle at the centre of the arc.

Similarly, the **area of a segment** is given by $\pi r^2\dfrac{x}{360}$.

3D shapes

Shape	Surface area	Volume
Cube/cuboid	Total area of all faces	*width* × *base* × *height*
Prism	Total area of both end faces and of faces running along length of prism	Surface area of one end face multiplied by length
Pyramid	Total surface area of all faces	(*base length* × *base width* × *height*) ÷ 3
Cylinder	$2\pi r^2 + (2\pi r \times length)$	$\pi r^2 \times length$
Cone	$\pi r(r + \sqrt{(height^2 + r^2)})$	$\pi r^2 \times (height \div 3)$
Sphere	$4\pi r^2$	$(4\pi r^3) \div 3$

Note that the formulae for a cone and sphere will be provided to you in the exam.

4.2 Vectors

Vectors provide us with information on the **magnitude** and **direction** of a movement from one point to another. Vectors may be symbolised as $\overrightarrow{XY}$ – this represents the vector going from a point, X, to another point, Y.

Vectors can be presented in this format $\begin{pmatrix} x \\ y \end{pmatrix}$ where x represents the distance travelled in a horizontal direction and y represents the distance travelled in a vertical direction.

A minus sign indicates that movement occurs in the opposite direction, so if $\begin{pmatrix} x \\ y \end{pmatrix}$ was designated as x units to the right, y units upwards, $\begin{pmatrix} -x \\ -y \end{pmatrix}$ would be x units to the *left* and y units *downwards*.

Vectors can be added together to give a resultant vector. Hence we could say that moving 3 units left and 4 units up, followed by 5 units right and 2 units down is equivalent to originally moving 2 units up and right because $\begin{pmatrix} -3 \\ 4 \end{pmatrix} + \begin{pmatrix} 5 \\ -2 \end{pmatrix} = \begin{pmatrix} 2 \\ 2 \end{pmatrix}$

If we move *against* a vector, we can indicate this by multiplying both numbers in the vector by -1. So going 2 units down and left is $-\begin{pmatrix} 2 \\ 2 \end{pmatrix} = \begin{pmatrix} -2 \\ -2 \end{pmatrix}$

4.3 Bearings

Three-figure bearings are used to describe a direction of travel in terms of the degrees of rotation *clockwise* from north.

Hence, having a bearing of 000 is the same as facing north; a bearing of 090 is the same as facing east; a bearing of 180 is the same as facing south; and a bearing of 270 is the same as facing west.

> **Top Tip:** Bearings can be used to construct geometric diagrams and solve problems. They should be treated like any other angle. Since they are always taken from the north, your knowledge of angles in parallel lines is particularly relevant.

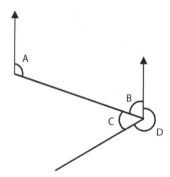

In the figure above, suppose we are told that the bearing A is 100 and bearing D is 230. If we were asked to find out C, we know that A + B = 180° (because co-interior angles add up to 180°) so B = 80°. Therefore B + D = 80 + 230 = 310°. So C must equal 50°.

5. Statistics

5.1 Presenting data

Bar charts

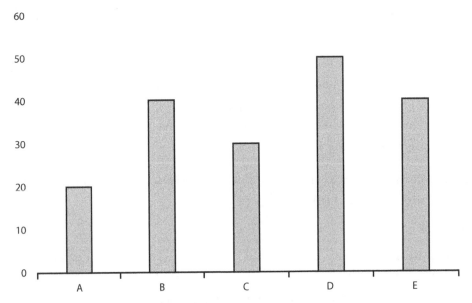

Used predominantly for presenting data that can be arranged into groups or categories. The length of the bar is proportional to the data represented.

Pie charts

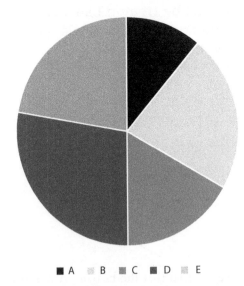

Used to display proportions of a whole. The size of a segment is related to the size of the proportion it represents.

Line graphs

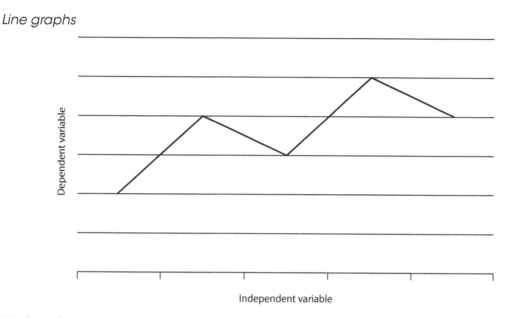

Used to observe general trends by joining up data points. Allows us to see how one variable is affected by another.

> **Top Tip:** As with *every* graph in the BMAT paper, whether it is in a physics, maths, chemistry or biology question, pay *very* close attention to the axes. Make a note of the labels (variables) on each axis. Sometimes examiners will give you a graph with a shape that you are familiar with (for instance, the rate of reaction line) but with differently labelled axes (they may put 'rate of reaction' on the *y*-axis as opposed to 'amount of product'). Make a careful note, too, of where points on the graph lie on the axes. Always check to see whether a point lies exactly in line with a labelled value on the axis, or whether it is in line with an unlabelled value just next to it.

Cumulative frequency graph

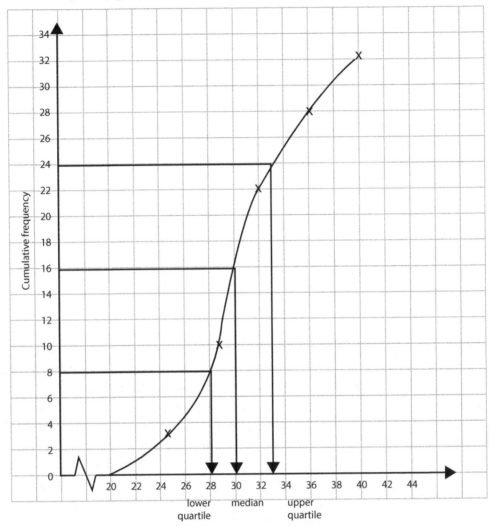

This graph shows the **running frequencies** of grouped data. Note that the *x*-coordinates of each point on the graph are placed at the **upper bound** of the group they represent. So if I was recording the frequency of people in different age groups, and one of my groups was for people between 10 and 20 years old, on the cumulative frequency graph I would mark the frequency of that age group by placing a point at '20 years old'.

It is easy to read the median, lower quartile and upper quartile values by using the cumulative frequency on the *y*-axis.

Box plots

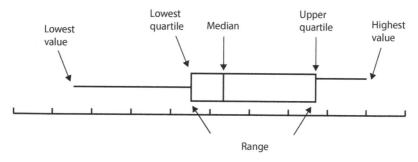

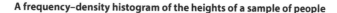

Box plots are also used to display certain statistics. The 'whiskers' of the box plot show the smallest and largest data points. The 'sides' of the box show the upper and lower quartiles, and the central line in the box shows the median value.

Histograms

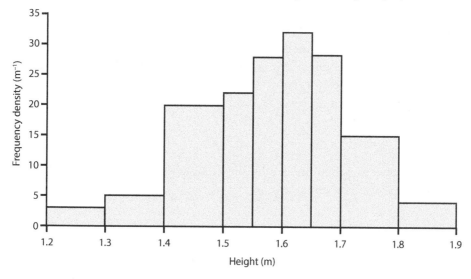

Histograms are used to represent the frequency of grouped data. They are particularly useful at showing the frequency of grouped data with groups of uneven width. **Frequency density** is the variable on the y-axis. The **area** of a bar on a histogram represents the **frequency** of data in that group.

Scatter diagrams

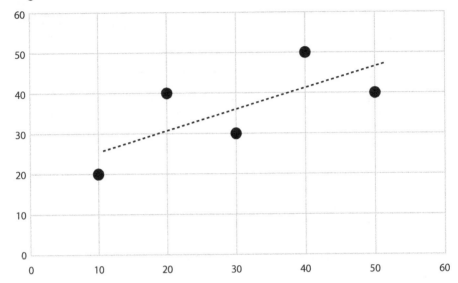

These are used to display relationships between two variables. Data points are placed at coordinates that correspond to the values on the *y*- and *x*-axes. The shape formed by the points on the graph provides information about the type of relationship between the variables (if any). A **line of best fit** may be used to display a trend.

5.2 Averages

Mean

The values are summed and then divided by the number of individual values. Incorporates all the data but may be skewed by outliers.

3, 4, 2, 1, 5, 6, 3, 1, 2

Total – 27

Mean – 27 ÷ 9 = 3

Median

The values are placed in ascending order and the 'middle value' is selected. If there are two middle values (i.e. in even datasets) the midpoint of these values is taken. The median is not skewed by outliers, but is time-consuming to calculate.

3, 4, 2, 1, 5, 6, 3, 1, 2

Ordered – 1, 1, 2, 2, 3, 3, 4, 5, 6

Middle value – 3

Lower quartile

The value that is one-quarter of the way through the dataset when the data is arranged in ascending order. If you divide the dataset into halves after working out the median, without including the median in the remaining numbers, the lower quartile is the median of the lower half of the dataset.

3, 4, 2, 1, 5, 6, 3, 1, 2

Ordered – 1, 1, 2, 2, 3, 3, 4, 5, 6

Middle value – 3

Lower half – 1, 1, 2, 2

Middle value of lower half – 1.5

Upper quartile

The value that is three-quarters of the way through the dataset when the data is arranged in ascending order. Similar to above, but the upper quartile is the median of the upper half of the dataset.

3, 4, 2, 1, 5, 6, 3, 1, 2

Ordered – 1, 1, 2, 2, 3, 3, 4, 5, 6

Middle value – 3

Upper half – 3, 4, 5, 6

Middle value of upper half – 4.5

Range and interquartile range

The differences between the lowest and highest values and the difference between the upper and lower quartiles respectively.

3, 4, 2, 1, 5, 6, 3, 1, 2

Difference between highest and lowest values – 6 – 1 = 5

Difference between the upper and lower quartiles – 4.5 – 1.5 = 3

Mode

The most common value in the dataset. If several values are equally common with the highest frequency, they are *all* modal values. The mode is not skewed by outliers, but it is not very representative of the dataset in its entirety.

3, 4, 2, 1, 5, 6, 3, 1, 2

Numbers appearing most frequently – 1, 2 and 3; all three are modes.

6. Probability

6.1 Probabilities of Single Events

The **probability** that a certain outcome, A, will happen is given by:

$$P(A) = \frac{\textit{total number of ways A could occur}}{\textit{total number of possible outcomes}}$$

This can be established **experimentally** by looking at the number of times A occurs in a set number of trials.

If an outcome is *certain* to happen, it has a probability of 1 (i.e. A is the only possible outcome).

If an outcome is *impossible* or *certain not to happen*, it has a probability of 0 (i.e. A is not a possible outcome).

Mutually exclusive outcomes of an event are ones which cannot occur together. If there are *only* two outcomes to an event, A and B, and they are mutually exclusive, the probability that either one will occur is:

$$P(A \text{ or } B) = P(A \cup B) = P(A) + P(B) = 1$$

That is, the probabilities of all the mutually exclusive outcomes of an event sum to 1.

The probability of an outcome, A, *not* happening is equal to

$$P(\text{not } A) = P(A)' = 1 - P(A)$$

6.2 Probabilities and Venn diagrams

Sometimes it is helpful to display probabilities using Venn diagrams.

Let us imagine we have two outcomes, A and B. These can be represented on a Venn diagram like so:

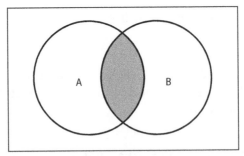

The probability that *all* these outcomes will occur, i.e. that A and B will occur, is equal to the **intersection** on the Venn diagram. Using Venn diagram notation we write:

$$P(A \text{ and } B) = P(A \cap B)$$

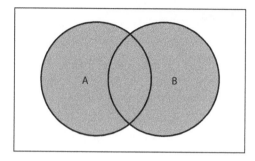

The probability that *any* or *at least one* of the events will occur is equal to the **union** of all sets on the Venn diagram:

$$P(A \text{ or } B) = P(A \cup B)$$

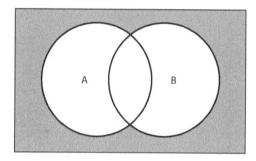

The probability that *none* of the events will occur is equal to region outside the sets:

$$P(\text{not } A \text{ or } B) = P(A \cup B)'$$

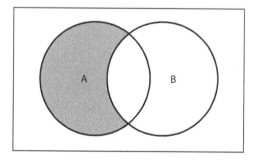

The probability of *just one* event occurring is equal to the set that represents that event minus the intersection with other events:

$$P(\text{just } A) = P(A) - P(A \cap B)$$

When outcomes are *not* conditional on each other, then the following are true:

$$P(A \cap B) = P(A) \times P(B)$$

$$P(A \cup B) = P(A) + P(B)$$

6.3 Conditional probabilities

Conditional probabilities of outcomes occur when one outcome is dependent on another outcome. A typical GCSE and BMAT example is picking coloured balls out of a bag in sequence without replacing them. Because the balls aren't replaced, the total number of outcomes possible changes each time you pick a ball, so the probability of picking any one colour keeps on changing.

When tackling these types of question, it is usually helpful to draw a tree diagram. In the tree diagram, we write the probability of a certain outcome at each branch point. To work out the probabilities of multiple outcomes we *multiply* moving along a branch and we *add* parallel branches.

Note that parallel branches represent mutually exclusive events.

As an example, if I had a bag with three red and two green balls inside, and I had to pick three balls from the bag without replacing them, I could draw this tree diagram:

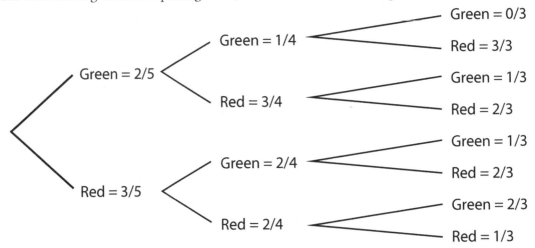

To find out the probability of picking a red ball, then a green ball, then another red ball, I just have to read along the relevant branches, multiplying as I go:

$$P\ (red\ then\ green\ then\ red) = \frac{3}{5} \times \frac{2}{4} \times \frac{2}{3} = \frac{12}{60} = \frac{1}{5}$$

The probability of picking a red, then green, then red *or* green, then red, then green is:

$$\frac{1}{5} + P\ (green\ then\ red\ then\ green) = \frac{1}{5} + \left(\frac{2}{5} \times \frac{3}{4} \times \frac{1}{3}\right) = \frac{1}{5} + \frac{6}{60} = \frac{3}{10}$$

The probability of an outcome, *A*, occurring **given that** another outcome, *B*, has already occurred can be worked out with the following equation:

$$P(A|B) = \frac{P(B \cap A)}{P(B)}$$

So the probability that a red ball is picked on the third go *given that* a red ball was picked on the second go is equal to the probability that a red ball is picked on the third go *and* a red ball was picked on the second go divided by all the probabilities that red was picked on the second go.

P (red picked on third go and second go) $= \left(\frac{2}{5} \times \frac{3}{4} \times \frac{2}{3}\right) + \left(\frac{3}{5} \times \frac{2}{4} \times \frac{1}{3}\right) = \frac{3}{10}$

P (red picked on second go) $= \left(\frac{2}{5} \times \frac{3}{4}\right) + \left(\frac{3}{5} \times \frac{2}{4}\right) = \frac{3}{5}$

P (red picked on third given picked on second) $= \frac{3}{10} \div \frac{3}{5} = \frac{1}{2}$

Top Tip: Remember that $P(B \cap A)$ does *not* equal $P(A) \times P(B)$ when A is conditional on B, or vice versa.

There is a full mock BMAT exam with science questions, including model answers, at the end of the book.

SECTION 3

Essay

Overview

In Section 3 of the BMAT, you are required to write a short essay. This is a test of your ability to understand a statement and to present coherent, well-thought-out arguments. You are expected to do this in a clear and concise way, before reaching a balanced conclusion.

In this chapter, we are going to suggest a formulaic approach to Section 3, ensuring that you hit the right length and timing while picking up high scores – each and every time.

Format of the section

BMAT Section 3 will see you presented with four statements. These are usually quotations, or opinions expressed as if they were facts. Beneath each statement will be instructions, which usually ask you to explain the statement, formulate an objective argument and express your opinion.

You are expected to write one essay, addressing one particular statement/quotation. Your essay must fit on one side of A4 paper, which will be provided. You are allowed to make notes on a separate sheet of paper.

This section of the BMAT examination is time pressured – but not intensely so. Writing one side of A4 is easy to do in 10 minutes or less. The challenge, therefore, comes in planning your arguments and counter-arguments in such a way that they can be efficiently translated into a fluent and articulate essay.

What is Section 3 testing?

According to the BMAT guidelines, 'this section tests ability to select, develop and organise ideas and communicate them in writing in a concise and effective way'.

Note that the words used here are all precise, analytical ones. There is no mention of creativity, flair or innovation – or any of those artistic adjectives that strike fear into the scientific minds of many prospective medics.

Don't confuse writing an essay with 'being creative'. Within your one side of A4, you want to appear logical, concise, reasoned and systematic. Basically, like a scientist.

Trying to be too creative isn't only a misunderstanding of the task. It is also an unnecessary risk. Creativity comes and goes, and depends upon inspiration. Analytical, systematic approaches can be reproduced with far less variance.

Our aim in this chapter is to equip you with a replicable methodology to ensure success in Section 3.

Top Tip: Don't try to be overly creative. Your approach should be more Charles Darwin and less Charles Dickens!

How is Section 3 marked?

Your essay will be marked on two things:

1. the quality of your content, and
2. the quality of your English.

Content is given a score between 1 and 5.

5 is the best mark; 1 is the lowest. When awarding a mark for content, examiners will be looking at the following:

- Has the candidate addressed the question in the way demanded?
- Have they organised their thoughts clearly?
- Have they used their general knowledge appropriately?

As with the summary of what the section is testing, take note of the types of words used here. The emphasis is always on relevance, clarity and organisation.

Many students worry about how they will be able to write a good essay if they don't know a lot about the subjects raised within the statements.

Don't worry!

Nowhere in the mark scheme does it say that you will be marked for your knowledge. It is a test of how you use what you know – not what you know per se. That said, it is fair to assume that having some knowledge of the topic will help you formulate strong arguments and showcase your technique.

An answer that scores an amazing 5 for quality of content should exhibit the following traits:

- All aspects of the question are addressed
- Excellent use of the material
- Excellent counter-proposition or argument
- The argument is cogent
- Clear and logical
- Breadth of relevant points
- Compelling conclusion

When practising writing essays, go through your responses with this list next to you and tick off the ones yours possesses.

Top Tip: Make sure you address all of the criteria from the mark scheme to score highly for content.

Quality of English is scored from A to E.

A is the best mark; E is the worst. Ultimately, the examiner is assessing whether you have expressed yourself clearly using concise, compelling and correct English.

An answer which scores an A for this should tick the following boxes:

- Fluent
- Good sentence structure
- Good use of vocabulary
- Sound use of grammar
- Good spelling and punctuation
- Few slips or errors

Your overall score will be a combination of a number (awarded for content) and a letter (awarded for quality of English). Your aim is to get an A5. Your paper will be marked by two examiners and your final score will be the average of the two. If there is a significant discrepancy between the scores given, then a third examiner will break the deadlock.

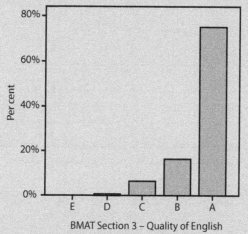

BMAT Section 3 – Quality of English

From this graph, you can see that most students score highly on their quality of English. Those who sometimes struggle are international applicants. If English is your second language, make sure you keep things simple and stick to vocabulary which you understand. It's also important that you practise writing in English and get your work checked by a native speaker.

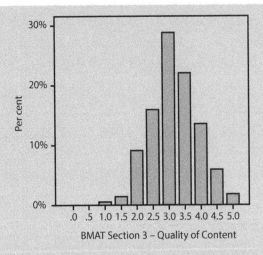

BMAT Section 3 – Quality of Content

This next graph shows typical scores for quality of content. You'll notice that these represent more of a bell-shaped curve. That means most students score in the mid-range, with few hitting top marks. The good news? This is where you can really stand out!

Question structure

The question structure in BMAT Section 3 is pretty uniform. You have to answer only one question out of four. Each question consists of a statement or quotation, followed by a series of prompts. These prompts will usually equate to:

1. Explaining the statement

2. Providing objective arguments

3. Reaching a balanced conclusion

In recent years, by far the most common question structure has been:

Statement or Quotation

Explain the statement. Argue to the contrary of / argue for the statement. To what extent do you agree with the statement / what is your opinion on the subject of the statement or quotation?

Note that this is based on analysis of the last few years of BMAT. It is not a cast-iron guarantee.

Top Tip: Prepare for the most common task structure but be ready to adapt to variations.

Your essay structure

Given the above, you can plan your essay quite precisely. That includes exactly how much you are going to write for each different section. This is important because you have a limited space on your one side of A4 – and you need to maximise it to fulfil all the criteria within the mark scheme.

So, we suggest adhering to the following guidelines:

Section	Sentences	Words
Explanation	1–2	20–40
Objective argument	5–8	130–180
Extent of agreement	5–8	130–180
Total:	11–18	280–400

Think about it for a minute. 11–18 sentences are not much at all. This is a double-edged sword, however. While it means you don't have to produce huge reams of fluent text in just half an hour, it also makes every single sentence crucial. You can't waste words!

So, you should start by being aware of sentence structure.

Sentence structure

Our advice on this is straightforward: keep it simple! Writing short, punchy sentences will ensure that you maximise clarity and impact. The last thing you want to do is start writing a long, meandering sentence which confuses the reader (and quite possibly yourself).

Here are two indicators that might suggest your sentences are getting too long:

1. They contain lots of fancy grammar or punctuation like semicolons. Elaborate use of grammar is probably unnecessary and could confuse the examiner – as well as yourself! Short, snappy sentences are preferable to long, meandering ones full of semicolons, which are often not needed and frequently misused.

2. They contain numerous conjunctions, like 'and' and 'but' in a single sentence. Consider the following two examples:

    a. It is important to practise BMAT Section 3 because it is one of the most challenging sections of the exam and offers a chance for candidates to stand out but it is also important to practise other sections of the exam and overall exam technique.

    b. It is important to practise BMAT Section 3 because it is one of the most challenging sections of the exam. It therefore offers a chance for candidates to stand out. However, it is also important to practise other sections of the exam, in addition to overall exam technique.

Which do you think is better?

We believe that option 'b' provides more clarity and a more discernible line of logical thought. You can see that the simple act of breaking things up into shorter sentences instantly adds cohesion. It is also easier and quicker to write like this!

> **Top Tip:** As you write each sentence, sound it out in your head. This will help you keep things clear and improve the fluency of your writing.

The statement/quotation

What kind of statement can you expect? Well, it will be no more than two or three sentences (it is often just one). It is often science- or medicine-related, though not 100% of the time. However, it won't be highly technical. That is, the statement won't relate to drug calculations or how to perform surgery!

Generally speaking, there are two types of statement:

1. An opinion stated as fact

In a world where we struggle to feed an ever-expanding human population, owning pets cannot be justified. (2013)

2. A quotation

'The art of medicine consists of amusing the patient while nature cures the disease.' Voltaire. (2011)

When deciding which one to tackle, make sure you select one which you understand perfectly. If you find any of the vocabulary or the syntax confusing, steer clear. Ideally, there might be one or two which you not only understand, but are actually interested in. This will help you formulate arguments for and against.

If you see something that you feel very strongly about, that might be helpful as you will have plenty to say. However, it is essential you still present a balanced essay which appreciates both sides of the argument and isn't aggressively partisan.

Explaining the statement/quotation

The first part of the task will almost always ask you to explain what the statement/quotation means. This can be phrased in slightly different ways. Over the last few years, we have seen all of the following:

- 'Explain what this statement means.'
- 'Explain what you think the above means.'
- 'What does the above imply?'
- 'What do you understand by the above?'
- 'Explain the argument behind the above.'

Ultimately, they are all asking the same thing: explain the statement!

Though this will only end up taking a couple of sentences, it is absolutely critical. The rest of the essay rests upon the foundation of your explanation. Any misunderstandings in your explanation are likely to be transmitted – and magnified – throughout your entire essay.

So, how do you go about explaining the statement? Well, we advocate three simple steps:

1. **Identify the key terms.** Key terms are the ones that stand out and really form the bones of the statement.

2. **Define these key terms.** In your notes, write what is meant by the key terms, without using the term itself. This doesn't need to be a dictionary definition, but should be as clear and objective as possible.

3. **Apply context and combine.** Fuse together these definitions so that they dovetail with one another and provide a cohesive overall meaning in one or two sentences.

Now let's explore three steps through a worked example, using the following quotation:

'A scientific man ought to have no wishes, no affections – a mere heart of stone.' Charles Darwin

Explain what this statement means.

Step one – identify the key terms

Which are the key terms that give the statement its meaning? In other words, which terms do you need to 'translate' to explain to someone, in a different (preferably simpler) way, exactly what Darwin is getting at? We would choose the following:

1. *'Scientific man'*

2. *'Ought'*

3. *'Wishes/affections'*

4. *'Heart of stone'*

Step two – define these key terms

Now that we have identified the key terms, we need to arrive at the best way of conveying their meaning. As mentioned above, this does not necessarily mean a dictionary definition. The idea should be to make it easily comprehensible, while accounting for the context. Do not try to impress by using overcomplicated language. Clarity is always the goal.

So:

1. *'Scientific man'*

    – Person seriously involved in scientific pursuits

2. *'Ought'*

    – Should/ideally

3. *'Wishes/affections'*

    – Emotional traits

4. *'Heart of stone'*

    – Metaphor for emotional detachment

Step three – apply context and combine

By fusing together the definitions above, we might arrive at the following explanation, which is clear, concise and effective:

'Charles Darwin is suggesting that a person who is seriously practising science would, in an ideal world, be completely free from emotion.' (21 words)

Please note that there have recently been some examples of BMAT essays that have asked you to 'explain the reasoning' behind the statement. In this case, you will need to adjust your approach slightly.

Our recommendation is to stick to the same three-step plan above, but to then add a layer of interpretation, in order to ensure that you are seen to be addressing the task precisely.

This additional content should go one step further, suggesting the rationale behind the statement. In the example above, for instance, we might add:

'The reasoning behind this statement might well be that, since science is by definition objective and precise, the fickle nature of human emotion is an obstacle to the discovery of scientific truth.'

Note two things here:

Firstly, we have specifically used the phrase 'the reasoning behind this statement' in order to flag to the examiner that we are addressing the task at hand.

Secondly, the use of the expression 'might well'. This is chosen because it is hard to know exactly what Darwin's reasoning was, without being able to ask him (a circumstance we consider unlikely!).

> **Top Tip:** Make sure you nail your explanation. Building an essay on top of a faulty explanation is like building a castle on sand!

Argue objectively

The second part of the task in Section 3 will almost always demand an objective argument. That can mean one of three things:

- Argue against ('to the contrary of') the statement
- Argue for the statement
- Argue both for and against the statement

The overwhelming favourite over the last few years has been 'argue to the contrary' of the statement.

When arguing 'to the contrary of the statement', you should try to come up with two or three arguments, each demonstrated by a clear example. We recommend noting these down as bullet points in your notes.

What they are looking for here is a breadth of arguments, clearly and logically articulated and supported with strong examples. Too many times, we see candidates approach the argument from only one angle, or use multiple examples to demonstrate a single point. Both of which will result in a failure to register top marks.

Again, let's consider 'argue to the contrary' with the aid of a worked example:

'The art of medicine consists of amusing the patient while nature cures the disease.' Voltaire

Argue to the contrary that medicine does in fact do more than amuse the patient.

Let's assume that we have already explained the statement as follows:

'Voltaire implies that the key skills involved in medicine are those that simply reassure or distract the patient, while their ailment corrects itself naturally over time.'

We have therefore equated 'amusing', in this context, with reassuring and distracting the patient. It is worth noting that we have not used the modern definition, which equates to making someone laugh. Remember: context is crucial and dictionary definitions are often misleading in this task.

So, three examples of situations where medicine does, on the contrary, do more than amuse the patient might be as follows:

- Emergency surgery – e.g. stent in coronary artery
- Faster healing – e.g. orthopaedic gamma nail
- Prescribing medication – e.g. HIV

This is how it would look in our notes section, with a prompt followed by an example. Then, when written onto the paper, it would read something like this:

Contrary to Voltaire's statement, there are many instances in which medicine does more than amuse the patient. This is often true of medical procedures that have been scientifically proven to physically improve patients' well-being faster, or more dramatically, than nature.

This is certainly the case in emergency procedures, such as the insertion of a stent into one of the coronary arteries of the heart in order to relieve an acute blockage to blood flow. It is also true of procedures which speed up healing, like the insertion of an orthopaedic gamma nail, which can realign a fracture of the lower limb with much faster and more consistent results than could realistically be expected to occur naturally.

Furthermore, a doctor is able to prescribe medications and treatments that can cure or contain illnesses that might progress if left to nature. One example is HIV, which requires prescribed medication to prevent it developing into AIDS.

(139 words)

It is important that you remember that at this stage of the task you need to argue objectively. Your personal opinion is not relevant – yet! That comes into play later, when you are (usually) asked to what extent you agree with the statement or quotation.

You should try to tailor your language accordingly. Words that lend themselves nicely to objective arguments are ones like:

- Therefore
- However
- In light of
- Consequently

- For example
- For instance

Phrases like 'I think' and 'in my opinion' are therefore not appropriate at this stage of your essay.

There is one other thing we would like to stress here. We have focused on 'arguing to the contrary' because that has been the most common request in the second part of Section 3 in recent years.

However, you may well get asked to 'argue for' a statement. In this case, it's not too difficult to adapt. Simply apply the above methodology, but note arguments 'for' rather than arguments 'against'.

As you are about to find out, you will ultimately need to argue both ways, anyway. Because when expressing the extent to which agree, you logically will have to balance any arguments against with arguments for, or vice versa!

To what extent do you agree?

The final part of the task usually prompts you to express an opinion. This is generally done by asking you the extent to which you agree with the statement/quotation, or by asking: 'to what extent do you agree that...' followed by a paraphrasing of the statement/quotation.

Let's remember that you will almost certainly have just put forward some objective arguments 'for' or 'against' (most likely 'against') the statement/quotation. Therefore, in order to conclude the extent to which you agree, it is a good idea to begin by counterbalancing those arguments.

In other words, if you just argued to the contrary, you will want to put forward some points in favour of the statement/quotation. Or, if you just argued in favour, you will want to make a case for the contrary standpoint.

Once you have done this, you will be well positioned to make a well-balanced conclusion. This should appreciate that there are merits to both sides.

You are dealing with statements and quotations that are contentious and complex. That is the nature of the task: to see how you grapple with them. In such cases, it won't simply be a case of falling one way or the other. The clue is in the question: 'to what extent...' You are expected to see shades of grey, not simply black and white.

> **Top Tip:** As a doctor, you will encounter patients from many different cultures, with many different perspectives. So being able to appreciate a variety of viewpoints is essential.

So, how do you begin the counterbalancing process? The first step will be to come up with some counter-arguments in your notes.

Let's continue with the Voltaire example. You will recall that the quotation was:

'The art of medicine consists of amusing the patient while nature cures the disease.' Voltaire

And the final part of the task asks:

To what extent do you think Voltaire is correct?

Given that we already provided arguments to the contrary, we should now think of two or three arguments in favour. These might be jotted into our 'notes' section as follows:

- 'Amusing' in this context can equate to 'listening to', or 'sympathising with', a patient
- There is an art to this
- Nature can cure many ailments (e.g. common cold)

And, after weighing these against our previous arguments to the contrary, we might reach a conclusion that, in note form, looks like this:

- In some conditions, the emphasis is on 'amusing' the patient while nature takes its course.
- In others, it is important to take actions proven to have a physical effect.

When writing up the counterbalancing arguments and the conclusion, we therefore end up with this:

Nonetheless, Voltaire's standpoint is not without merit. In this context, 'amusing' the patient can be taken to mean 'offering sympathy' or 'reassuring' them.

There is clearly an art to this and it is extremely valuable in medicine. For example, in the case of the common cold, there is little a doctor can do to help medically. But the doctor can reassure the patient that there is nothing seriously wrong, and that they will be well again soon.

Overall, there are some times when the best thing a doctor can do is to 'amuse', or 'reassure', a patient while nature takes its course. At other times, though, medical procedures or prescriptions must be administered to prevent an illness progressing.

Perhaps we can conclude that the best doctors are those who combine the 'art' of sympathy and reassurance with the 'science' of swiftly applying necessary physical procedures.

(144 words)

There are a few things that you should note here.

The first is that we presented both sides of the argument before concluding. The second is that though we have reached a conclusion (this is essential if you are to gain full marks for fulfilling all the requirements of the question) it is not a partisan one. It simultaneously concludes while appreciating the nuances involved.

You will also see that the type of language has shifted. Having put forward an objective argument in objective terms, we now see words like 'overall', 'at other times' and 'perhaps'. This is now the language of subjectivity and compromise. By saying 'we can conclude that...' or 'in conclusion' we are flagging to the examiner that we have recognised and fulfilled this part of the criteria.

On that note, good words to use in this part of the task include:

- Perhaps
- Maybe
- Nonetheless
- On the other hand
- Overall
- On balance
- In conclusion

> **Top Tip:** Use clear wording to demonstrate to the examiner that you are fulfilling the mark scheme criteria. 'On the other hand...' highlights that you are introducing a breadth of points; 'in conclusion' stresses that you are coming to an overall conclusion.

Diagrams

On the cover sheet of Section 3, you are told that you can use diagrams 'if they enhance communication'. Our stance on this is that, generally speaking, we don't recommend it. There are a couple of reasons for this.

The first is that it is an unusual tactic. That is not to say that it is a bad one. No doubt, it could work wonderfully well. However, we feel that it is higher risk. The examiner might love it, but they also might be thrown off. Our approach to Section 3 is about following a clearly defined methodology that reduces variance in performance and outcome. Therefore, using diagrams does not sit well with us.

The second reason we don't particularly favour diagrams is that they potentially take up a lot of space. As we know, you only have one side of A4, so space is a premium asset in this task. Remember, it is called an essay writing task. Again, if we think about the risk profile, you are using a considerable percentage of your real estate here.

In addition, diagrams often aren't easy to draw. So if you make a mistake and need to start again, you might end up wasting a valuable portion of your answer sheet.

None of this is to say that using diagrams prohibits you from scoring highly in BMAT Section 3. It just means that it is not the approach we prefer when championing a methodology which will consistently reach the top marks.

Timing: step-by-step approach

So, you've reached the final part of your BMAT exam. The clock has just started ticking; you now have half an hour to finish Section 3. What exactly do you do, step by step, minute by minute?

The big news is that we advocate that you do not touch your final answer sheet until you have spent 15 minutes writing notes.

> **Top Tip:** Stick to the notes section until you have planned your essay; the answer sheet is for writing up a plan, not freestyling!

Here is the procedure we suggest you follow:

Step 1: Choose your question (2 minutes)

Read all the options carefully. Choosing the right one of the four to tackle is important. There are certain criteria you should be looking for here.

In terms of the statement/quotation, you want one that you are certain you understand fully. This is non-negotiable!

Any doubt about the terminology used or the meaning intended should be a major red flag. You also want a statement/quotation about which you know something, or for which arguments for and against spring to mind. This is highly preferable.

Then there is the task itself. What exactly are they asking you to do?

As we have said, asking you to explain, argue against and explain the extent to which you agree is the most common format over the last three years. But there are numerous variations. If you have prepared for the most likely scenario and two follow this pattern, perhaps those are better options than the two that don't. Whatever you do, do not assume the task instructions will follow the most common template: read them carefully.

We feel that you can weigh up the options and choose your question in two minutes.

Step 2: Explain it: notes (3 minutes)

It is highly likely that the first part of the task will ask you to explain the statement/quotation. So, in your notes, write down the key terms and jot down definitions next to each. Remember, these aren't dictionary definitions, but ones which simplify within context. Then knit these into a clear one- or two-sentence explanation, ready to transcribe straight onto your answer sheet.

Remember to add a line about the 'reasoning behind' the statement/quotation if this has been requested by the question.

We believe that this can be done in three minutes.

Step 3: Argue objectively: notes (5 minutes)

Next, you will be asked to argue for or against the statement – most likely against (or 'to the contrary' as it tends to be phrased). So, you will need to write three arguments, in bullet point form, in your notes section. Include an example next to each one.

As you write each point, try to start thinking about how it will be developed when writing it up. When it comes to doing so, you can either use two or three points, depending on space. So start with your best!

Step 4: To what extent: notes (5 minutes)

Now you want to write two or three more bullet point arguments for the opposite position. So, if you argued to the contrary above, jot down some arguments for the statement/quotation now.

Then, think of a short conclusion and write this down. Your essay needs to finish powerfully, so any crossing out and moving around should be done here in your notes first.

Step 5: Write it! (15 minutes)

The last 15 minutes should be spent writing up your notes into a clear, cogent essay on the answer sheet. Fifteen minutes is a long time to write one side of A4, so there's no need to rush or be frantic. You should keep your handwriting neat and think about what you are writing. However, do still keep an eye on the clock!

Final Tips: Here are our final tips for success on BMAT Section 3:

- Read questions carefully.
- Use short sentences.
- Use clear vocabulary.
- Sound it out as your write it – this will promote fluency.

Mock BMAT exam and answers

Below is a full mock BMAT exam, followed by worked answer solutions. You should allow yourself a two-hour window to sit the exam. We recommend that you take a break after the exam, and only work through the answers once rested!

You should allow yourself the following timings:

- Section 1: 1 hour

- Section 2: 30 minutes

- Section 3: 30 minutes

To help simulate the exam experience we have created sample computer-read mark sheets for you to use. Visit our website to print these in advance: www.themedicportal.com/bmatbook.

You must not use a calculator, dictionary or any other electronic device.

Good luck!

Section 1

Instructions to candidates:

There are 35 multiple choice questions to be answered in one hour. Each question is worth one mark and there is no negative marking. Download and print the computer-read mark sheet from our website (www.themedicportal.com/bmatbook), and use a soft pencil to complete.

You may use the exam paper to perform rough work and calculations. Calculators are not permitted.

START

1. The four digits of the PIN number for my debit card are such that their numerical sum is the same as their numerical product. The first letter of each digit, when written in order as words, can be used to form the word FOOT.

   What is the total number of letters required to spell the first, second and last digits?

   A. 9

   B. 10

   C. 11

   D. 12

   E. 13

   F. 14

2. I have five glasses of equal shape and size. I know the following facts:

- Glass A contains a third of the amount of water as Glass C.
- Glass B contains as much water as the water in Glasses D and E combined.
- Glass C contains as much water as the water in Glass A and half the water in Glass E combined.
- Glass D contains a fifth of the total volume of water.

Which of the following statements is correct?

A. Glass B contains the most water.

B. Glass A contains more water than Glass D.

C. Glass B contains the average amount of water.

D. If the total volume of water in the glasses was 1250 ml, E would contain 125 ml of water.

E. Glasses B and D combined contain more than half the total amount of water.

3. In the Middle Ages, thousands of women were famously tried and executed for crimes of witchcraft. However, it is a myth that the majority of these were executed because they had a form of mental illness or were unpopular locally. People in the Middle Ages were in fact reluctant to classify someone as a witch. When this happened, it meant that the woman in question had to be removed from society, for the benefit of herself and the community. She therefore had to be supported for the remainder of her life by her fellow citizens. This could often be a costly process, and one which people preferred to avoid whenever possible. This shows the paradoxical nature of the Middle Ages, where superstition and pragmatism were intertwined in a way that is unfamiliar today.

What conclusion can be drawn from the argument in the passage?

A. Witchcraft trials were gender-driven, with the victims almost always women.

B. Women who were found guilty of witchcraft faced swift execution after their trial.

C. The Middle Ages was not a time of pure individualism.

D. The Middle Ages was characterised by superstition and pragmatism in equal measure.

E. Today we live in a less superstitious society than was typical in the Middle Ages.

4. A group of 50 medical students are discussing which medical field they would like to enter:

- 17 say they are considering entering oncology.
- 25 say they are considering entering ophthalmology.
- 29 say they are considering entering obstetrics and gynaecology.
- 5 say they are considering only oncology.
- 4 say they are considering either oncology or obstetrics and gynaecology.
- 1 says she is considering all three.

How many are considering either oncology or ophthalmology?

A. 5

B. 6

C. 7

D. 8

E. 9

5. In 2006, England introduced a smoking ban which made it illegal to smoke in all enclosed work places in the country. The ban, which was largely popular at the time, was the result of increased understanding of the dangerous effects of passive smoking, whereby those in near proximity to smokers can suffer adverse health effects. However, the decision to sign into law a blanket ban on all enclosed smoking has been met with increased opposition in recent times. And it is true that the law is fundamentally undemocratic. If people want to smoke, they should be able to, since it is their body, at the end of the day. A pressure group called 'Freedom to Choose' has recently launched a campaign for a judicial review of the legislation, claiming that the law is a violation of human rights.

Which of the following best describes a flaw in the above argument?

A. The purpose of laws is that they supersede the wants of the individual.

B. Smoking can cost society money in NHS bills.

C. Smoking affects the health of more than just the person doing it.

D. It is difficult to enforce a smoking ban if it is not total.

E. The ban cannot be undemocratic as it was popular when introduced.

6. An airline awards reward points to its most frequent customers according to the following formula:

2 reward points for every hour flown + 10 reward points for every country visited = total number of reward points

David and Stuart both have 70 reward points. If David flew for twice as many hours as Stuart and visited 5 countries, how many countries must Stuart have visited?

A. 2

B. 3

C. 4

D. 5

E. 6

7. A signalling system depends on the rotation of parts which can be viewed as two-dimensional shapes.

The shapes are all aligned such that one straight edge on one shape is parallel with a straight edge on an adjacent shape. When a shape on the left rotates clockwise, this forces the shape to its right to rotate anticlockwise. Similarly, if the left shape rotates anticlockwise, the adjacent shape rotates clockwise.

Shapes rotate until a new pair of edges are parallel, for example:

If the leftmost triangle rotates clockwise, the square will rotate anticlockwise and the rightmost triangle will rotate clockwise.

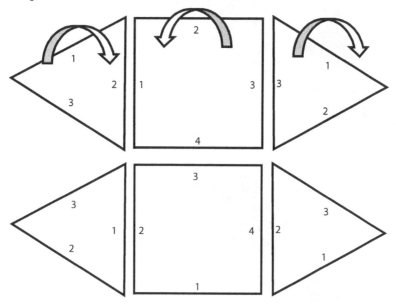

The signalling system has the following arrangement of shapes, and the leftmost shape is rotated clockwise once:

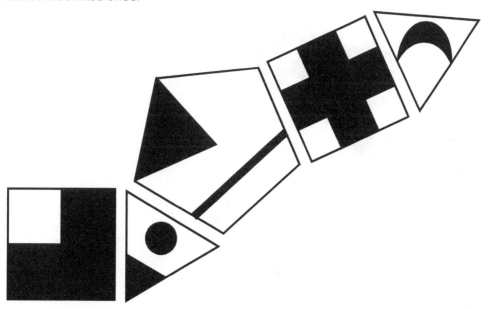

Which of the following arrangements represents the shapes after their rotation?

A.

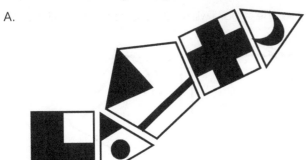

B.

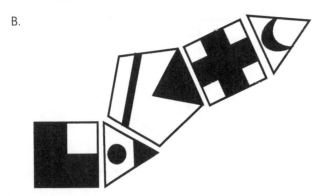

C.

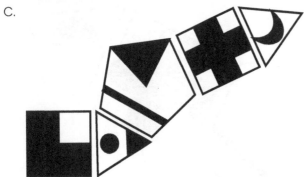

D.

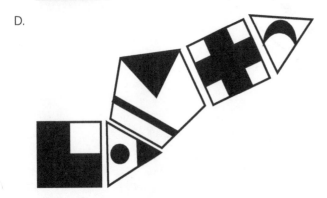

E.

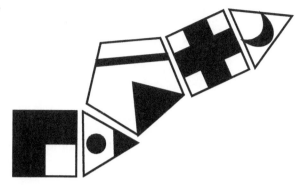

8. Most people will tell you that the 'value' of something is how much someone is willing to pay. Therefore, when people complain that top footballers are 'paid too much', what they are saying makes no sense. The fact that someone is willing to pay such wages, without being coerced or unfairly influenced, proves that they are paid sufficiently. Even leading economists fall into this trap. Often, after a major economic incident, economists state that the subsequent price crash reveals that certain products were 'overvalued'. But this cannot be the case. The value only fell because it had been created by investment from the past. If a product was not truly 'worth' a certain amount, it would not achieve this value in the first place.

    Which of the following best describes a weakness in the above argument?

    A. It ignores the fact that value is subjective.

    B. It fails to differentiate between 'good' value and 'bad' value.

    C. It confuses 'value' and 'worth'.

    D. It refers to only extreme examples.

    E. It treats a subjective premise as objective.

9. A teacher wants to find out how many pupils in her GCSE Maths class passed their exams with grades A*–C. She constructs the following table:

	Set 1	Set 2	Set 3	Set 4	Set 5	Total
A*	19	10	5	1	0	35
A	5	14	13	5	1	38
B	4	14	24	16	6	64
C	0	6	10	20	24	61
Total	28	44	53	42	31	198

    After she draws the table, she notices one of the individual entries in the table has been typed incorrectly.

    Which value is incorrect?

    A. Set 1, Grade B

    B. Set 1, Grade C

    C. Set 2, Grade A*

D. Set 2, Grade C

E. Set 3, Grade A

F. Set 3, Grade C

G. Set 4, Grade A*

H. Set 5, Grade B

I. Set 5, Grade C

10. A mathematician has the following algorithm in which he can input any number to produce a new number:

1. Multiply your number by 10

2. Subtract 5

3. If the number is odd, multiply by 2. If the number is even multiply by 3

4. Subtract 10

He inputs a number and receives the output 30. However, later that day, he notices he had forgotten to do step 4.

What was his original number?

A. 1.9

B. 2

C. 2.5

D. 3

E. 10

F. 15

11. One of the most widely misunderstood phrases in popular culture must surely be: 'the survival of the fittest'. Generally, Darwin's mantra is taken to refer to physical strength, with the implication being that nature is tough and only has room for the fiercest of survivors. This, though, is misguided. In fact, the phrase should be understood to mean the 'survival of the best-suited'. Let's consider an example. The kiwi bird cannot fly. And, when approached by predators, it simply remains stationary and makes no sound. Yet, the fact the species continues to reproduce and exist in the wild makes it an effective survivor, on par with lions and great white sharks.

Which of the following, if true, would weaken the argument presented?

1. Many more kiwi birds are kept as pets in comparison to those that live in the wild.

2. While lions and sharks live on multiple continents, there are no kiwi birds in any countries outside of New Zealand.

3. Scientists believe that over 10,000 flightless bird species have become extinct in the last million years.

A. 1 only

B. 2 only

C. 3 only

D. 1 and 2 only

E. 1 and 3 only

F. 2 and 3 only

G. None of the statements

12. My four children are called Fiona, Ben, George and Darwin. Their birthdays are on the 15th, 35th, 144th and 323rd days of the year respectively.

    Which two of my children have their birthday on the same day of the week?

    A. Fiona and Ben

    B. Fiona and George

    C. Fiona and Darwin

    D. Ben and George

    E. Ben and Darwin

    F. George and Darwin

13. Every Tuesday night at the university union is quiz night. There are a total of 30 questions, with every correct answer scoring 8 points, but 3 points are deducted for every incorrect answer. Team A entered the quiz, answering every question and scored 152 points.

    How many correct answers did Team A get?

    A. 8

    B. 11

    C. 19

    D. 20

    E. 22

14. Here is a net that can be assembled into a cube:

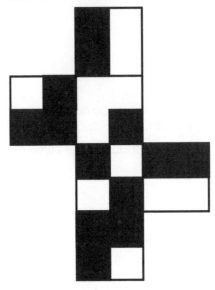

Which of the following are possible representations of the cube?

A.

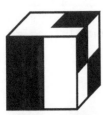

B.

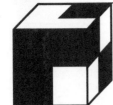

C.

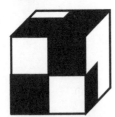

D.

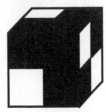

E.

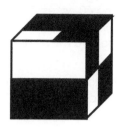

A. A and B

B. B and C

C. D and E

D. C and E

E. D and A

15. Many people fear unemployment, not only due to the insecurity of having a limited income and lack of purpose in life, but also due to the social stigma that can be attributed to not having a job. But, in the 21st century, graduates fear not unemployment but *underemployment*. Underemployment refers to an individual working in a position for which they are overqualified. As a result, they receive lower wages, are less stimulated and become easily frustrated. In many cases, underemployment is seen as less desirable than unemployment. Therefore, the percentage of graduates employed represents an example of an anachronistic statistic which can be too easily skewed by those in underemployment. Academic institutions should take this into account to provide more accurate statistics.

What is an assumption made in the above argument?

A. Unemployment and underemployment are effectively the same.

B. Only university graduates can be underemployed.

C. Underemployment has only become an issue in the 21st century.

D. Underemployment is measurable.

E. Statistics from academic institutions are unreliable.

16. A scientist is preparing for an experiment. He must dilute every 1 part of concentrate with 4 parts of water. By mistake, he added 300 cm³ water to 25 cm³ concentrate.

What must he add to the resulting mixture to obtain the correct concentration?

A. 50 cm³ of water

B. 100 cm³ of water

C. 200 cm³ of water

D. 3 cm³ of concentrate

E. 50 cm³ of concentrate

F. 75 cm³ of concentrate

G. 100 cm³ of concentrate

17. Mary plans on hosting a charity coffee morning and plans on baking 60 cakes. She makes the cakes in batches of 12. Each batch takes 20 minutes to prepare and 15 minutes to cook in the oven (during which time she can begin to prepare the next batch).

Once the cakes have finished baking they require 5 minutes to cool slowly, during which time the oven is occupied and cannot be used for baking. Once the cooling period is finished the oven is ready for use again.

If Mary starts at 15:00, at what time will she finish, assuming she doesn't take a break?

A. 16:40

B. 17:00

C. 17:15

D. 17:20

E. 17:30

F. 17:40

18. A spy needs to get from the north side of a fortified wall to the south side. He can only do this by passing through a gate on the north side of the wall, followed by a gate on the south side of the wall.

North side

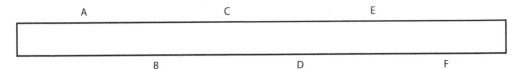

South side

The gates are guarded; however, guards are obliged to take rest breaks. When a guard is resting, the spy can slip by unnoticed. The spy knows the following rules apply to the guards' rest breaks:

- At least one guard must be resting on each side (north and south) of the wall.
- No two guards at adjacent gates (e.g. A and B, B and C, C and D, etc.) can both be resting at the same time.
- The spy cannot go through a gate where a guard is resting if it lies between (i.e. is adjacent to) two gates where the stationed guards are both awake.

Which of the following statements are true?

1) If a guard is awake at A, the spy may be able to escape through Gate F on the south side.

2) If a guard is resting at E, the spy will not be able to cross the wall.

3) If a guard is awake at E, the spy will be able to escape.

4) Only an even number of guards may be resting at any time.

A. 1 only

B. 2 only

C. 2 and 3

D. 3 and 4

E. 1 and 2

F. 1, 2 and 3

19. The health secretary, Jeremy Hunt, has stated that by 2020 he would like to see at least half of the country's 40,000 consultants work regular weekends. Currently, the consultants have the right to opt out of weekend work. However, such an opting out is detrimental to our health service: consultants, who are doctors with the highest levels of experience, are likely to be better at identifying and treating rare medical complications than their more junior colleagues. Therefore if consultants are lacking in hospitals at the weekend, patients' lives will be endangered. Indeed, this is borne out by certain statistics that show, for example, that a patient is 15% more likely to die when admitted on a Sunday rather than a Wednesday. For these reasons, the health secretary's statement should be applauded.

Which of the following statements, if true, would strengthen the above argument?

A. All consultants have postgraduate qualifications in medicine.

B. Consultants would have anticipated that they would be expected to make certain sacrifices at the outset of their medical careers.

C. The increase in mortality at the weekend is found to be predominantly due to rare medical complications that went unnoticed.

D. Senior doctors in other countries work regular weekend shifts.

E. The presence of consultants boosts the morale of junior doctors.

20. I decide to go for a walk. I start by facing north. I then perform the following movements:

- I walk 10 metres forward, then I turn right by 35°.
- I walk 15 metres forward, then I turn right by 90°.
- I walk 5 metres forwards, then I turn left by 45°.
- I turn around to face the opposite direction, then I walk 20 metres forward.
- I do these previous four steps once again, in the same order.

Between which directions am I now facing?

A. North and east

B. South and east

C. North and west

D. South and west

E. Due south

F. Due west

21. Faisal runs a small business and regularly has to send packages to local companies. A local courier company charges a flat rate per pick-up with an additional fee per kilometre travelled.

   - Delivering a package to the station, which is 4 kilometres away, costs Faisal £10.
   - Delivering a package to the cinema, which is 3 kilometres away, costs Faisal £8.60.

   How much would it cost Faisal to send a package to the sweet shop, located 5 kilometres away?

   A. £5.80

   B. £11.40

   C. £12.50

   D. £23.40

22. Joseph played a game at the fair. He had to take out 2 balls from a bag of 50 balls. There were balls of different colours in the bag. Both the balls he picked were black. The man running the stall said:

   'There was a 4/175 chance that you would do that.'

   What is the maximum number of red balls that could have been in the bag at the start?

   A. 46

   B. 42

   C. 38

   D. 34

   E. 27

23. In 2008 the world witnessed arguably the worst financial disaster in history. Part of the problem which engulfed the world economy was that large financial institutions all over the world had amassed huge liabilities, which far outweighed their own assets. In fact, prior to the crash, many confidently predicted that certain organisations were 'too big to fail'. While large proportions of debt usually create fear of default, advocates of this theory asserted that the level of debt and amount of money involved in some cases was so vast that governments couldn't afford to let this happen. They had a shock when American mortgage companies Freddie Mac and Fannie Mae were allowed to go to wall, soon followed by 158-year-old investment bank Lehman Brothers.

   Which of the following is a conclusion that can be drawn from the passage above?

   A. Large liabilities always lead to a situation of economic difficulty.

   B. The government was surprised by the failure of Freddie Mac.

   C. The sense of security propagated by advocates of 'too big to fail' was paradoxical.

   D. The 'too big to fail' theory had not existed prior to 2008.

   E. Company age does not protect a company from failure.

24. A regular convex polyhedron (Platonic solid) has 20 vertices, 30 edges and an unknown number of faces.

What is the name of the shape?

A. Hexahedron

B. Heptahedron

C. Octahedron

D. Nonahedron

E. Dodecahedron

25. In a factory, workers can assemble either 10 large toys or 25 small toys in 1 hour. Assuming they have only 3 hours to assemble an order of 100 large toys and 500 small toys, how many workers do they need?

A. 10

B. 15

C. 20

D. 25

E. 30

26. The table below shows the mean systolic blood pressure of four ethnic groups (Caucasian, Afro-Caribbean, South Asian, Oriental Asian) measured in a student-led research experiment, along with the statistical error bars:

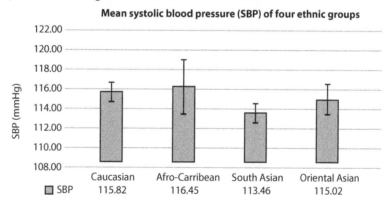

Mean systolic blood pressure (SBP) of four ethnic groups

	Caucasian	Afro-Carribean	South Asian	Oriental Asian
SBP	115.82	116.45	113.46	115.02

Based on this graph, which of the following statements is true?

A. Oriental Asians have the lowest mean systolic blood pressure.

B. There is no significant difference in the mean systolic blood pressure between the four ethnic groups.

C. Afro-Caribbeans have the highest systolic blood pressure among the four ethnic groups.

D. There is a significant difference in systolic blood pressure between Caucasians and Oriental Asians.

E. South Asians have the lowest systolic blood pressure.

27. History teaches us that prohibition rarely works. It famously failed in the United States when alcohol was banned there in the 1920s. The amount of alcohol consumed did not decrease and prohibition resulted in a dramatic increase in violent crime, motivated by the illicit rewards available from bootlegging. There is now a similar situation in the United States when it comes to recreational drugs. Prohibition has failed to prevent the consumption of these drugs, despite the fact that they are illegal. Violent crime prevails as a result, as gangs fight for lucrative territory. Therefore, legislators should learn lessons from the past and end the 'prohibition' on drugs, thereby solving the majority of these issues.

What is an assumption made in the above argument?

A. Recreational drugs and alcohol carry the same health risk.

B. Socially, drugs are viewed the same way now as alcohol was in the 1920s.

C. Violence can only be solved by removing prohibition.

D. People are more likely to consume a product if it is illegal.

E. Legislative decisions have significant consequences.

28. In a school, the test results from two physics exams were recorded by the teacher as follows:

	Test 1	Test 2
Lyla	64	67
Jacob	65	78
Kerry	79	67
Lolly	82	40
Connard	20	25
Dilayla	23	23
Eric	24	63
Frodo	27	61
Germaine	41	72
Hina	42	65
Anna	10	8
Ben	12	88

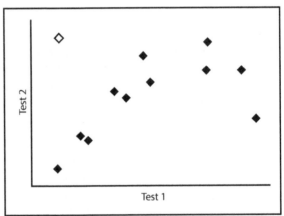

Which student's test results are represented by the white diamond?

A. Ben

B. Dilayla

C. Eric

D. Frodo

E. Germaine

F. Hina

G. Anna

29. I am thinking of installing solar panels. The cost of installation is high; however, in the long term I will be able to recoup the money through the savings I make on my annual energy bills, which will be reduced to zero. My energy bill remains constant, year to year.

    In addition, I will be able to sell any surplus electricity back to the national grid at 10 pence/kWh.

    In the first year of having solar panels, I predict I will have recouped a total of 5% of the original installation cost of the solar panels, and that I will sell 5000 kWh of energy back to the grid.

    In the second year of having solar panels, I predict that I will have recouped an *overall* total of 11.25% of the original installation cost of the solar panels, and that I will sell 7500 kWh of energy back the grid.

    What was the installation cost of the solar panels?

    A. £20,000

    B. £25,000

    C. £60,000

    D. £70,000

    E. £200,000

30. The graphs below show how the speed of four different cars, S, T, U and V, vary with time over a period of 20 seconds:

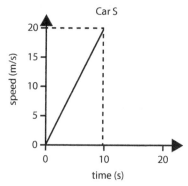

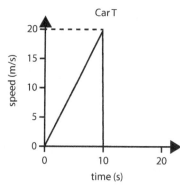

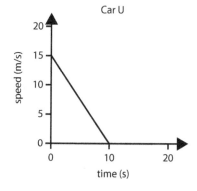

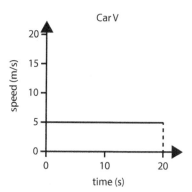

At the end of the 20-second period, Car V continues at a constant speed for an additional 40 seconds. Car S, however, travels at a constant speed from 10 seconds onwards for another 50 seconds.

After 60 seconds, what is the difference in distance travelled between Car S and V?

A. Car S travelled 800 m further than Car V.

B. Car V travelled 800 m further than Car S.

C. Car S travelled 1400 m further than Car V.

D. Car V travelled 1400 m further than Car S.

E. Car S travelled 900 m further than Car V.

F. Car V travelled 900 m further than Car S.

31. In 2012, a ruling from the European Court stated that car insurance companies could no longer adjust their rates based on a person's gender. Before this, it was often the case that women received lower rates due to the fact that, statistically, young male drivers are much more likely to suffer a crash that leads to serious injury or death. According to recent statistics, there is less of a difference between men and women when it comes to the frequency of minor collisions. However, the ruling is still fundamentally unfair because careful female drivers are now effectively subsidising their young and reckless male counterparts.

Which of the following, if true, would most weaken the argument in the passage?

A. A car crash often involves two cars and the insurance company usually is unable to determine the genders of both drivers involved in the incident.

B. It is possible to sometimes drive carefully and sometimes drive recklessly.

C. Before the ruling, insurance companies would add a large premium to all males' policies, effectively subsidising female drivers.

D. There is little correlation between the seriousness of traffic accidents and the premiums charged by the insurance company.

E. There is little statistical divergence between the likelihood of being involved in a serious accident and gender in people over 35.

32. There are currently 480 workers in a hospital: 55% are nurses and 20% are doctors. One hundred more workers are hired, which results in 55% of the workers being nurses and 20% doctors.

How many new doctors and nurses are hired?

A. 20

B. 55

C. 75

D. 100

E. 118

33. A laboratory uses an 11-digit reference code when processing blood samples.

The first three digits of the code represent the clinic code, the next six digits represent the clinic date (written as dd/mm/yy) and the final two digits are a security code. The security code is calculated as the clinic code – clinic day. If the security code has more than two digits, it's divided by 10 and the resultant number rounded.

One of the blood tests from the laboratory has the code: 12527120398.

Which of the following codes could be from the same laboratory?

A. 12419030211

B. 12532111593

C. 12508161412

D. 12522031512

E. 12526101499

34. I am given three candles, each of which, when lit, will burn for exactly 20 minutes. It is possible to light both ends of each candle.

Assuming I have three candles, which of the following time periods (in minutes) can I measure through lighting candles?

A. 5, 10, 15, 20, 30, 60 and 90 minutes

B. 20, 40 and 60 minutes

C. 10, 15, 20, 30 and 60 minutes

D. 10, 20, 30, 40 and 60 minutes

E. 10, 15, 20, 30, 60 and 70 minutes

35. In the Western world, the concept of polygamy is seen as completely alien to the values that should be adhered to in society. In cultures which have a long tradition of marriage for life to one spouse, the idea of being married to more than one person simultaneously is seen not only as illegal, but also morally wrong. Yet, in many other parts of the world polygamy is accepted for the exact reasons for which it is rejected in the West. In these (usually poorer) communities, families in which a husband has more than one wife can provide economic security and enhanced social status for a greater number of people. So, polygamy is viewed there as a positive, rather than a negative, domestic dynamic.

Which of the following best describes the aim of the above passage?

A. To highlight the difficulty of applying moral judgement on a global scale

B. To explain the limitations of marriage in the Western world

C. To argue against the idea that polygamy is wrong

D. To defend an action that is universally seen to have negative results

E. To evaluate which situations are suited to polygamous relationships

Section 2

Instructions to candidates:

There are 27 multiple choice questions to be answered in 30 minutes. Each question is worth one mark and there is no negative marking. Download and print the computer-read mark sheet from our website (www.themedicportal.com/bmatbook), and use a soft pencil to complete.

You may use the exam paper to perform rough work and calculations. Calculators are not permitted.

START

1. The diagram below shows the expression pattern for a disease in a single family. Currently, the status of Individual A is unknown. What are the chances that individual A will also have the disease in the scenarios given in the table below?

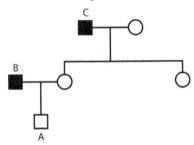

	Individuals B and C are heterozygous	Individual C is homozygous
A	50%	100%
B	50%	0%
C	50%	50%
D	100%	50%
E	0%	50%

2. Which of the following statements about polymerisation are true?

A) Organic molecules that act as the monomers in polymerisation will also decolourise hydrogen bromide.

B) Monomers must be saturated hydrocarbons.

C) C_2H_3OH, C_3H_6 and $C_2H_4Cl_2$ are all potential monomers.

A. A only

B. B only

C. C only

D. A and B

E.   B and C

F.   A, B and C

G.   None

3. If 3.6 dm³ of carbon monoxide gas is reacted with iron (III) oxide according to the equation below, what is the mass of iron that will be produced?

(one mole of any gas at room temperature and pressure has a volume of 24 dm³; A_r: C = 12, O = 16, Fe = 56)

$$3CO + Fe_2O_3 \rightarrow 2Fe + 3CO_2$$

A.   56 g

B.   12.6 g

C.   5.6 g

D.   126 g

E.   1.26 g

4. Sodium-22 is a radioactive isotope of sodium (atomic number: 11). It emits *positrons* as a type of beta decay (positrons are the positively charged antimatter counterpart of electrons). It has a half-life of approximately two and a half years.

Which of the following statements about sodium-22 is correct?

A) If we have one mole of sodium-22, after five years we will be left with 5.5 g of sodium-22.

B) When sodium-22 decays, the difference between its new atomic number and its atomic mass is 10.

C) The decay product of sodium-22 is likely to have a violent reaction with fluorine gas.

A.   A only

B.   B only

C.   C only

D.   A and B

E.   B and C

F.   A, B and C

5. Make a the subject of:

$$P = 1 - \sqrt{\frac{n^2 + a}{n + a}}$$

A. $a = \dfrac{n(1+P)^2 - n^2}{(1 - (1+P)^2)}$

B. $a = \dfrac{n(1-P)^2 - n^2}{(1 - (1-P)^2)}$

C. $a = \dfrac{n(1-P)^2 - n^2}{(1-P)^2}$

D. $a = \dfrac{n(1-P)^2}{(n-(1-P)^2)}$

E. $a = \dfrac{n(1-P)^2 + n^2}{(1+(1-P)^2)}$

6. A patient has 5 litres of blood. They need to be given a drug intravenously such that the final concentration of the drug in their blood is 0.1 mmoldm^{-3}. If the relative molecular mass of the drug is 300, what mass of the drug needs to be added to an IV bag containing 500 cm³ of fluid?

(Assume that the drug is not broken down in the body for the duration that the patient is on the IV drip, and that the patient does not lose any fluid.)

A. 0.15 g

B. 0.165 g

C. 15 g

D. 16.5 g

E. 165 g

7. Which of the following statements are true?

A. Ligase cuts genetic material at a specific point.

B. Treatment for diabetics can be produced on a large scale by inserting the bacterial insulin gene into crops.

C. Insulin can be inserted into bacterial plasmids using enzymes.

D. A human cell may contain four copies of a single gene.

E. Increasing temperature of ligase indefinitely will increase its catalytic activity indefinitely.

8. Two objects, A and B, are identical in mass. They are both held in a vacuum chamber 5 m above the ground. They are then dropped at different times such that at time t, object A is 4 m above the ground and object B is 3 m above the ground.
(Assume $g = 10$ ms^{-2}).

What is true of the objects at time t?

A. Object B has a slower velocity than object A.

B. Object B has 33% more potential energy than object A.

C. Object B has lost more energy as heat, due to the effects of drag, than object A.

D. Even if the mass of the objects was known, the kinetic energy of each object could not be established without further information.

E. The velocity of object B is greater than that of object A by a factor of $\sqrt{2}$.

9. Identify the letters a, b, c and d by balancing the equation below:

$$aH_2SO_4 + bHI \rightarrow H_2S + cl_2 + dH_2O$$

	a	b	c	d
A	1	8	4	4
B	2	8	4	8
C	1	4	8	4
D	1	4	4	8
E	2	4	8	8

10. The function $f(x)$ is represented by the line $y = 2x^2 + 3$.

    Which of the following statements are true?

    1) $f(x)$ crosses the line $y = x + 3$ at (0,3)

    2) The line $y = 2x^2 - 4x + 5$ can be written as $f(x - 1)$

    3) The line $y = 2x^2 - 4x + 5$ represents a translation of $f(x)$ by – 1 along the x-axis

    A. 1 only

    B. 2 only

    C. 3 only

    D. 1 and 2

    E. 2 and 3

    F. All three

11. Which statement could describe a possible part of the sequence of neuronal signalling in a reflex arc?

    A. Effector tissue → motor neuron dendrite → sensory neuron axon

    B. Sensory neuron axon → receptor tissue → sensory neuron dendrite

    C. Interneuron axon → motor neuron dendrite → motor neuron axon

    D. Sensory neuron axon → Interneuron axon → Interneuron dendrite

    E. Sensory neuron dendrite → sensory neuron axon → receptor tissue

12. I have some tea I would like to keep hot. What sort of container should I put it in?

    A. A container made of metal, with a shiny interior and a matt exterior

    B. A container made of wood, with a matt interior and a matt exterior

    C. A container made of metal, with a shiny interior and a shiny exterior

    D. A container made of wood, with a shiny interior and a shiny exterior

    E. A container made of wood, with a shiny interior and a matt exterior

13. A substance has an empirical formula of C_2OH_4. Its M_r is 88.

When reacted with calcium carbonate, it forms a salt, water and carbon dioxide. When reacted with ethanol it forms an ester. What could be the name of the substance?

(A_r: C = 12, O = 16, H = 1)

A. Propanoic acid

B. Butanoic acid

C. Propanol

D. Ethanoic acid

E. Butanol

14. The concentration of calcium ions in extracellular fluid is approximately 1 mmolL^{-1}. The concentration of calcium ions in the cytoplasm is approximately 0.1 µmolL^{-1}.

Under normal physiological conditions, protein X moves calcium ions out of the cell.

Which of the following statements is incorrect?

A. If a cell is placed into distilled water, calcium ions will move out of it against their concentration gradient.

B. If a cell is placed into 2 mmolL^{-1} calcium ion solution, the amount of energy in the cell consumed by protein X is likely to rise.

C. If a cell is placed into a 0.01 µmolL^{-1} calcium ion solution, water will move into the cell by osmosis.

D. If a cell is placed into distilled water, water will move into the cell by osmosis.

E. The extracellular concentration of calcium is 10,000 times greater than the internal concentration.

15. I have a bag filled with nine balls. Three are red, three are blue and three are green.

- If I pick a red ball, I get to pick again (unless I picked a blue ball previously).
- If I pick a blue ball, I am allowed to pick out one more ball and then I have to stop.
- If I pick a green ball, I have to stop without picking out any more balls.

What is the probability that I will pick out two red balls and a *single* ball blue (note – these do not have to be the only balls I take out)?

A. 3/56

B. 1/56

C. 1/28

D. 3/28

E. 1/1568

16. Which of the following statements is **not** true of sound waves:

   A. An object moving towards a loudspeaker at a constant speed will encounter sound waves at a higher frequency than those being produced by the loudspeaker.

   B. If the speed of sound is taken to be 330 m/s and the speed of light is 300,000 km/s, a sound wave of frequency 1650 Hz will have a longer wavelength than infrared radiation of frequency 30 GHz.

   C. A sound wave is longitudinal; therefore a sound wave travelling through air will cause air molecules to undergo a net displacement from their original positions that is parallel to the direction in which the wave is travelling.

   D. Sound waves above the human threshold of hearing can be utilised to provide a safer alternative to X-rays for medical imaging.

   E. A loudspeaker moving away from a stationary person will produce a sound with a higher tone than the sound that is perceived by the person.

17. Which of the following statements regarding the diagram below is true?

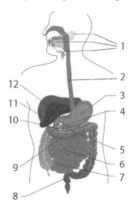

   A. The substance produced by structure 1 contains the enzyme salivary protease.

   B. The substance secreted by the walls of structure 3 plays an important role in the adaptive immune system.

   C. Structure 2 is maintained by C-shaped rings of cartilage.

   D. Structure 6 receives chyme from the duodenum.

   E. Structure 11 secretes bile into structure 12.

18. My younger brother is a keen mycologist. He is growing a patch of fungus in his room.

   - On day 1, the patch had an area of 5 mm^2.
   - On day 2, the patch had an area of 7 mm^2.
   - On day 3, the patch had an area of 12 mm^2.
   - On day 4, the patch had an area of 20 mm^2.
   - On day 5, the patch had an area of 31 mm^2.

What will the size of the patch be at the end of the month (day 30)?

A. 1281 mm²

B. 1333 mm²

C. 1457 mm²

D. 1600 mm²

19. Observe the circuit below:

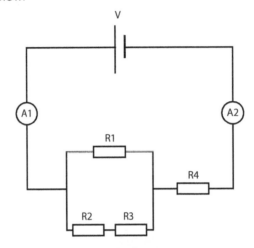

A1 and A2 represent the readings of two ammeters, and R1 to 4 represent the resistances of four fixed resistors. V is the voltage across the cell.

Which of the following statements are true?

A) A1 = A2 = V ÷ (R1 + R2 + R3 + R4).

B) This graph represents the relationship between resistance and voltage across R4:

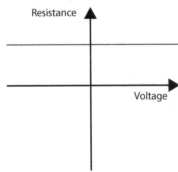

C) Multiplying R4 and A2 will give the amount of work done on each unit of charge that passes through the resistor in joules.

A. A only

B. B only

C. C only

D. A and B

E. B and C

F. A and C

G. A, B and C

20. Study the chemical equation below:

$CuSO_4 + Zn \rightarrow ZnSO_4 + Cu$

Which of the following statements are true?

A) The equation above shows the reduction of copper, which can also be summarised in the ionic half equation $Cu^{2+} \rightarrow Cu + 2e^-$

B) A copper anode, when placed in a solution of the copper compound shown in the equation above, will increase in size if a voltage is applied.

C) If carbon can be used to displace zinc from its compounds, carbon will also displace copper.

A. A only

B. B only

C. C only

D. A and B

E. B and C

F. A and C

G. None

21. A patient has an inherited disorder which means that her red blood cells are less effective at carrying oxygen than in a healthy person. The patient's father and brother have the condition, but her mother does not.

Which of the following statements are likely to be true?

A) The disorder is due to a mutation in a gene on the Y-chromosome.

B) The patient will have elevated levels of lactate in her blood compared to a healthy individual, following a period of anaerobic exercise.

C) The patient's blood pH will remain elevated for longer than in a healthy individual, following a period of anaerobic exercise.

A. A only

B. B only

C. C only

D. A and B

E. B and C

F. None is true

22. A concrete block weighs 50 kN. It is pushed at a constant speed across a horizontal surface between two points, A and B. While it is being pushed, it encounters a friction force of 40 kN (assume air resistance is negligible). The bulldozer that pushes the block expends 1 MJ of **useful** energy between A and B.

What is the distance between A and B?

A. 20 m

B. 25 m

C. 200 m

D. 250 m

E. 2.5 km

23. Hydrogen reacts with nitrogen to form ammonia. The reaction is reversible. When ammonia is produced, the reaction is exothermic. The graph below shows the production of ammonia (y-axis) over time (x-axis).

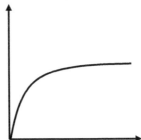

How will the same graph look (assuming the values on the axes stay the same) if a nickel catalyst is added and the temperature of the reaction system is increased?

A.

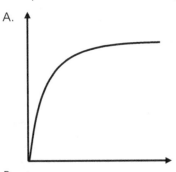

B.

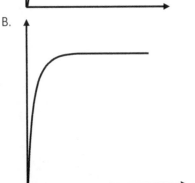

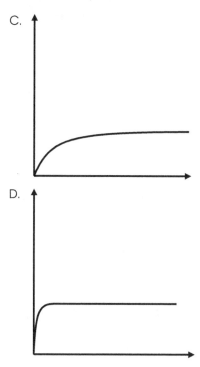

C.

D.

24. In a sixth-form college there are two biology classes. There are x students in class 1 and y students in class 2. In a recent test, the average score across the two classes was T. However, three highest-scoring students from class 2 were later discovered to be cheating, and their scores were later removed from the total. A new average, M, was established from the remaining marks.

If the average score of the cheating students was a, which of the following statements will definitely be true?

A) $M > a$

B) The median score will not change after the removal of the cheaters' scores.

C) $M = \dfrac{T(x+y) - 3a}{(y+x-3)}$

A. A only

B. B only

C. C only

D. A and B

E. B and C

F. A and C

G. All are definitely true

25. Which of the following substances would **not** be produced either as a result of the nuclear fission chain reaction of uranium-235 *or* the nuclear fusion of hydrogen?

A. Three free neutrons

B. Uranium-236

C. Heat energy

D. Deuterium

E. Krypton-90

F. Helium-3

26. Three nutrient mixtures were combined with either one of three preparations of digestive enzymes or saline solution preparation.

The nutrient mixtures were tested for the presence of glucose, glycerol and amino acids before and after the addition of the enzyme preparations. They were *only* tested for these chemicals.

The table below shows the results:

Nutrient mixture	Preparation used	Nutrients identified BEFORE addition of preparation	Nutrients identified AFTER addition of preparation
A	1	Glucose	Glucose
B	1	Glucose	Glucose, Glycerol
C	1	None	Glycerol
A	2	Glucose	Glucose
B	2	Glycerol	Glycerol
C	2	None	None
A	3	Glucose	Glucose
B	3	Glycerol	Glycerol, Amino Acids
C	3	None	Amino Acids
A	4	Glucose	Glucose
B	4	Glycerol	Glycerol
C	4	None	Glycerol

Which of the following statements *must* be true?

A. Preparation 3 is the saline solution.

B. Nutrient Mixture A does not contain starch.

C. Nutrient Mixture B contains all three of starch, fat and protein.

D. Nutrient Mixture C contains at least two different types of nutrient.

E. Protease in Preparation 3 digested another enzyme that was also in the preparation.

27. Which of the following statements is incorrect (assume $g = 10$ ms^{-2})?

    A. An accelerating object may move at a constant speed.

    B. A decelerating train on straight rails will not have a constant speed.

    C. An object falling at terminal velocity may have a net horizontal force acting on it.

    D. The work done on an object with constant acceleration is proportional to its mass.

    E. An object of mass 10 g falling towards Earth will reach terminal velocity when a drag force of 100 N acts upon it.

Section 3

Instructions to candidates:

Below are two writing tasks for you to practise. In the real BMAT exam, you will have a choice of four tasks but will only be expected to answer **one**.

Your answer must fit on one side of A4 paper. Download and print a replica Section 3 answer sheet from our website (www.themedicportal.com/bmatbook).

You can make preliminary notes. **Candidates with permission to use a word processor must not exceed 550 words**.

The tasks each provide an opportunity for you to show how well you can select, develop and organise ideas and communicate them effectively in writing. Diagrams, etc. may be used if they enhance communication.

You have 30 minutes to complete one task. Dictionaries and calculators may NOT be used.

1. 'The medical profession, after all, deals partly with guess work; we do not deal in absolutes.' Paul Beeson, MD

Explain what this statement means. Argue that there are times when the medical profession does deal with absolutes. To what extent do you agree that the medical profession deals partly with guesswork?

2. 'A man who cannot work without his hypodermic needle is a poor doctor. The amount of narcotic you use is inversely proportional to your skill.' Martin H. Fischer

Explain the argument behind this statement. Argue to the contrary, that the use of narcotics does not suggest a lack of medical skill. To what extent do you agree that being able to work without a hypodermic needle is the sign of a skilful doctor?

Answers

Below you will find an answer key for each section summarising the correct answers. There is also a sample score conversion, converting each score into a suggested BMAT score. This score is for guidance purposes, and allows you to see and compare performances. You can then review detailed answer explanations for each question, including sample notes and essays for section 3.

Section 1

Answer Key:

Question	Answer
1	B
2	E
3	C
4	C
5	C
6	E
7	C
8	E
9	F
10	B
11	G
12	C
13	E
14	D
15	D
16	E
17	B
18	B
19	C
20	B
21	B
22	B
23	C
24	E

Score Conversion:

Total Score	Suggested BMAT Score
0	1.0
1	1.0
2	1.0
3	1.0
4	1.0
5	1.0
6	1.3
7	1.8
8	2.1
9	2.5
10	2.8
11	3.1
12	3.4
13	3.6
14	3.9
15	4.1
16	4.4
17	4.6
18	4.8
19	5.0
20	5.3
21	5.6
22	5.9
23	6.2

Answer Key:

Question	Answer
25	A
26	B
27	E
28	A
29	A
30	A
31	D
32	C
33	E
34	C
35	A

Score Conversion:

Total Score	Suggested BMAT Score
24	6.5
25	6.8
26	7.1
27	7.4
28	7.7
29	8.1
30	8.5
31	9.0
32	9.0
33	9.0
34	9.0
35	9.0

1. Answer = B

We are given that the first letters of each digit, when written as words in order, spell FOOT. The only single digit that begins with O is 1 – therefore the second and third digits of the PIN must be 1.

For the first digit, F, the only options are 4 (four) or 5 (five), and similarly for the last digit, T, the only options are 2 (two) or 3 (three).

We know that the numerical sum is the same as the numerical product. This is only true if the first digit is 4 and the last digit is 2 (as $4 + 1 + 1 + 2 = 8$ and $4 \times 1 \times 1 \times 2 = 8$).

We can therefore deduce that the total number of letters required to spell the first, second and last digits is 10 (four, one and two).

2. Answer = E

This question requires you to work through each answer option in turn to assess whether or not it is correct. Based on the statements you know that:

$A = C/3$

$B = D + E$

$C = A + E/2 = C/3 + E/2$

$D = 1/5$

$B = 1/5 + E$

$6C = 2C + 3E$

$4C = 3E$

C = 3E/4

A = E/4

So A = E/4, B = 1/5 + E, C = 3E/4, D = 1/5, E = E

E/4 + 3E/4 + E + 1/5 + 1/5 + E = 3E + 2/5

3E + 2/5 = 1

E = 1/5

So A = 1/20, B = 2/5, C = 3/20, D = 1/5, E = 1/5

Assessing each answer option in turn:

A. Incorrect: C contains the most water

B. Incorrect: D contains more than A

C. Incorrect: B contains twice the average amount of water

D. Incorrect: E would contain 1250/5 = 250 ml

E. Correct: 2/5 + 1/5 = 3/5 which is greater than 1/2

3. Answer = C

The fact that suspected witches were exiled for 'the benefit of herself and the community' shows that people in the Middle Ages acted, at least in part, with the needs of a wider community in mind. This demonstrates that it was not a time of 'pure individualism'.

A is incorrect because while witches are always referred to as female in the passage, this does not mean that their trials were driven by gender.

B is incorrect because for people to worry about the cost of maintaining women guilty of witchcraft for the rest of their lives, it follows that they were not always executed 'swiftly'.

D is incorrect because while the passage says that superstition and pragmatism were intertwined, it does not say they existed in 'equal measure'.

E is incorrect because the passage does not say that we are less superstitious today – just that superstition and pragmatism are less intertwined.

4. Answer = C

This question can be answered using a Venn diagram. We are trying to work out area 'D'. We know that there are 50 students; however, the numbers for each subject add up to 17 + 25 + 29 = 71. Therefore, 71 – 50 = 21 must be due to students being counted more than once (i.e. the intersecting area on the Venn diagram).

Area G has been counted three times, so it must have been counted two more times than necessary. We know from the information given that this is equal to 1 (the one student considering all three subjects), so it must have contributed 2 × 1 = 2 to the extra counts. Therefore we know that the other overlapping areas, which have been counted one extra time each, must add up to 21 – 2 = 19.

We know that one of the overlapping areas, D, is equal to 4 (from the information we are given). We also know from the given information that A = 5.

So A + E + G + D = 17 or 5 + E + 1 + 4 = 17

So 10 + E = 17

Therefore E = 7

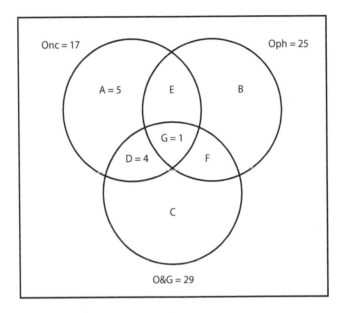

5. Answer = C

The argument states that 'the law is fundamentally undemocratic' and that people should be able to smoke based on the premise: 'it's their body'. But this is a flawed premise, because it is not only their body – we are told within the same argument that passive smoking impacts the health of others.

None of the other options directly removes or destabilises the main premises of the argument.

6. Answer = E

David's points can be calculated as:

- (David's hours × 2) + (10 × 5) = 70
- (David's hours × 2) = 20
- (David's hours) = 10

Therefore Stuart flew for 5 hours (as David flew for double the amount of hours). From this it is possible to calculate the number of countries he visited:

- (5 × 2) + (10 × number of countries) = 70
- (10 × number of countries) = 60
- (Number of countries) = 6

7. Answer = C

Markers indicate how the shapes move. Remember, a shape rotating one way induces a rotation in the opposite direction in the shape to its immediate right – a shape rotates until its edge is parallel with the edge of the adjacent shape.

So, going shape by shape:

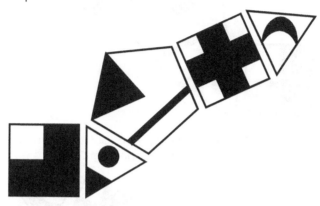

Becomes this, as the leftmost square rotates clockwise

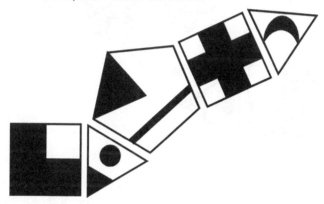

Which induces the triangle to rotate anticlockwise

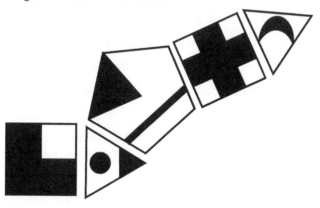

Which induces the pentagon to rotate clockwise

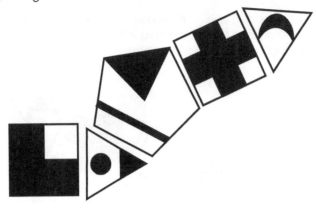

Which Induces the other square to rotate anticlockwise (but it looks the same), which in turn induces the triangle to rotate clockwise. This is arrangement C.

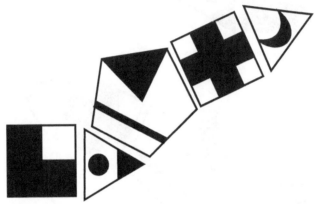

8. Answer = E

The argument starts by saying that 'most people will tell you that the value of something is how much someone is willing to pay'. This definition is subjective. But the argument treats it as a key, objective premise.

A is incorrect because this point is neither ignored nor weakening to the argument.

B is incorrect because while this is true, it does not reveal a weakness in the argument.

C is incorrect because, while both terms are used, they are not 'confused'.

D is incorrect because the examples can't be clearly identified as extreme.

9. Answer = F

Adding all the rows for each set, we find that the total for Set 3 (5+13+24+10 = 52) is different from its row total of 53. So one of the entries for Set 3 is incorrect.

Adding all the totals for each Grade row shows us that the problem is with Grade C. It should total 61 but only totals 60.

Hence Grade C for Set 3 must be the incorrect entry.

10. Answer = B

The important thing to notice is that in step one, we multiply by 10. This means that when we subtract 5 in step 2, the number will always be odd. Hence we can use the algorithm backwards (ignoring step 4):

- 30/2 = 15
- 15 + 5 = 20
- 20/10 = 2

So the mathematician's original number was 2.

Note: If you are not sure how to approach this sort of question, you could always look at the answers available and plug them into the algorithm.

11. Answer = G

None of the above statements would weaken the argument that the kiwi bird's continued ability to reproduce makes it an effective survivor on a par with the other animals cited.

1 does not weaken the argument because the premise given is that the bird still reproduces and exists 'in the wild', and this is not altered by the fact it is also kept as a pet on a wide scale.

2 does not weaken the argument because the ability to survive in multiple countries is not necessary an effective measure of survival skills.

3 does not weaken the argument because it refers to a general trend that may not be relevant to this specific case.

12. Answer = C

To work out which of the four children share their birthday on the same day of the week, the difference between the two birthdays should be divisible by 7.

Fiona's birthday is on the 15th and Darwin's birthday is on the 323rd. The difference between these two numbers is 304 which is divisible by 7. Therefore, Fiona and Darwin have their birthdays on the same day of the week.

13. Answer = E

Start by allocating correct answers = X and incorrect = Y. Therefore they scored 8X – 3Y = 152

We know they answered 30 questions, therefore X + Y = 30. We can multiply by 3 to give 3X + 3Y = 90

Add the two equations: 8X – 3Y = 152 and 3X + 3Y = 90

This gives 11X = 242 which is X = 22.

14. Answer = D

Questions asking you to construct three-dimensional shapes from two-dimensional templates are tricky. Work your way through each answer option in turn, finding analogous positions on the two- and three-dimensional shapes to compare. If combinations don't work, eliminate that option as well as other answer combinations containing that option.

In this question only shapes C and E can be assembled.

15. Answer = D

The argument states that 'the percentage of graduates employed represents an example of an anachronistic statistic' and that academic institutions should take underemployment into account 'to provide more accurate statistics'. For this to be possible, the number of underemployed students would need to be somehow measurable.

A is incorrect because the argument highlights differences between the two, rather than assuming them to be the same.

B is incorrect because the argument does not say that underemployment is exclusively a graduate problem.

C is incorrect because the argument does not state that underemployment is a unique issue of the 21st century.

E is incorrect because the argument states that these particular statistics are anachronistic rather than 'unreliable'. Nor does it make a judgement on other types of statistics from academic institutions.

16. Answer = E

The ratio of concentrate to water should be 1:4. The scientist's mixture of concentration to water has a ratio 25:300. This simplifies to 1:12.

So for every 1 part of concentrate, there is an extra 8 parts of water. There is 25 cm³ of concentrate, so there are 8 × 25 = 200 extra parts of water.

200/4 = 50 cm³ of concentrate needed to obtain the correct concentration.

17. Answer = B

You know that each batch takes 20 minutes to prepare followed by a 20-minute oven phase (as although the cooking time is 15 minutes, the cooling period during which the oven is in use is 5 minutes). During this oven period Mary can be preparing the next batch.

As Mary requires 60 cakes and can prepare them in batches of 12, she will need to bake 5 batches.

It will therefore take Mary 20 minutes to prepare the first batch, after which while each batch is cooking the next can be prepared. It will therefore take Mary 120 minutes to prepare and cook 5 batches, meaning she will finish at 17:00.

18. Answer = B

You need to assess each statement in turn to see if the spy can escape.

Statement 1: There are 2 possible configurations, neither of which the spy can escape in (as the gates with resting guards are between gates with awake guards). This is therefore false.

Statement 2: With a guard resting at E there is only 1 possible configuration, making it impossible for the spy to cross. Therefore this statement is true.

Statement 3: The spy cannot escape with this configuration so the statement is false.

Statement 4: There can be an odd number of guards resting. Note it can't be 1 because then only one side would have a resting guard and it can't be 5 because that would leave adjacent gates with resting guards, hence the odd number must be three with at least one guard on both sides. The statement is therefore false.

The only statement that is true is statement 2.

Configurations for each scenario:

Statement 1 – Option 1

A Awake		C Awake		E Resting
	B Resting		D Awake	F Awake

Statement 1 – Option 2

A Awake		C Resting		E Awake
	B Awake		D Awake	F Resting

Statement 2

A Awake		C Awake		E Resting
	B Resting		D Awake	F Awake

Statement 3

A Resting		C Awake		E Awake
	B Awake		D Resting	F Awake

Statement 4

A Resting		C Resting		E Awake
	B Awake		D Awake	F Resting

19. Answer = C

The summary of the argument is that consultants have the most medical experience and are better at identifying and treating rare complications; so when they are not there, patient lives are endangered; therefore, consultants should not be able to opt out of working at weekends.

A is incorrect because this is simply a reiteration of the statement 'Consultants, who are doctors with the highest levels of experience', except it is less informative because it doesn't tell us anything about the qualifications held by other doctors!

B is incorrect as this does not strengthen the argument that this particular 'sacrifice', i.e. giving up the weekend opting out, is necessary.

C is correct because this strengthens the premise that patients' lives will be 'endangered' if the chance of recognising/treating rare complications is reduced – hence it strengthens the whole argument.

Although D may be true, we are not told about the effect of this on patient mortality/well-being, and the argument hinges on that factor.

Again in E we don't know what effect this has on patient mortality, so it cannot be said to strengthen the argument.

20. Answer = B

Note, this is a question about bearings; the information regarding the distances is not needed to answer the question. Let us consider that, if I start facing north, if I rotate myself by 360° I will still be facing north. Therefore, I just need take into account how many degrees over a multiple of 360° I have rotated overall. By focusing on right turns, it is clear that I have rotated:

- 35 + 90 + (360 – 45) + 180 + 35 + 90 + (360 – 45) + 180 =
- 2 × (35 + 90 + (360 – 45) + 180) =
- 2 × 620 =
- 1240° to the right

Note that a turn 45° to the left is equal to a 360 – 45 = 215° degree turn to the right, in terms of final orientation.

This is equal to 3 × 360° + 160°, so in effect I have rotated 160° to the right from my original orientation. If I was originally facing north, therefore, I must now be facing between south (180°) and east (90°).

21. Answer = B

We can write the information given in terms of algebraic equations:

- Equation 1: $x + 4y = 1000$
- Equation 2: $x + 3y = 860$

Where x represents the flat rate and y represents the rate for each kilometre travelled.

We can then solve simultaneously by subtracting equation 2 from equation 1 giving us: $y = 140$ p. Plugging y back into either of equation 1 or 2 will give us $x = 440$ p. Hence the flat rate for pick-up is £4.40 and the rate for each kilometre travelled is £1.40.

So to deliver to the sweet shop would cost the flat rate pick-up of £4.40 plus 5 × £1.40 = £11.40.

22. Answer = B

Let n be the number of black balls in the bag. We know that $n/50 \times (n – 1)/49 = 4/175$

In other words, $n(n – 1)/2450 = 4/175$

$n(n – 1) = 9800/175$

$n(n-1) = 56$

$n^2 - n - 56 = 0$

$(n-8)(n+7) = 0$

So $n = 8$

For the maximum number of balls, we must assume that red and black balls were the only balls in the bag, so the number of red balls is $50 - 8 = 42$

23. Answer = C

This is because the passage states that while high proportions of debt usually lead to default, advocates of 'too big to fail' believed that very high proportions of debt reduced the risk of this happening in some cases. This represents a paradoxical situation, and therefore C is correct.

A is incorrect because the argument does not present enough information to evaluate if large liabilities 'always' lead to economic difficulty.

B is incorrect because 'advocates' were shocked, rather than the government.

D is incorrect because the argument does not discuss anything prior to 2008.

E is incorrect because, even though the age of Lehman Brothers is given, this is not related to protection from failure. It also does not preclude the fact that an even older company, or perhaps a much younger company, could have indeed been protected by age.

24. Answer = E

This question can be done using trial and error, assessing each answer option in turn. However, it would be faster to use Euler's formula: $F + V - E = 2$. (F = number of faces, V = number of vertices and E = number of edges)

Therefore, $F + 20 - 30 = 2$

$F = 12$

25. Answer = A

If you only had 1 hour, you would need 10 workers to assemble 100 large toys, and 20 workers to assemble 500 small toys = 30 workers.

As you have 3 hours, you require $30 / 3 = 10$ workers.

26. Answer = B

The error bars show the confidence intervals of the data. In this case, there is no statistical difference in systolic blood pressure between any of the groups, so none of statements A, C, D or E can be inferred. Statement B is therefore correct.

27. Answer = E

If legislative decisions – like ending prohibition on drugs – are to solve the 'majority of these issues', it stands to reason that they must have 'significant consequences'. But, since this is not demonstrated in the passage, it is an assumption underlying the argument.

A is incorrect because the argument is not concerned with the health risks of either substance.

B is incorrect because the argument is not concerned with how the substances are/were viewed socially.

C is incorrect because the argument does not assume that this is the 'only' way to reduce violence.

D is incorrect because the argument does not consider the reasons behind why people consume substances.

28. Answer = A

Using the graph you can see that the white diamond represents the highest score for Test 2 and the second-lowest score for Test 1. By using the table you can see that Ben came both top of Test 2 and second to bottom of Test 1.

29. Answer = A

The amount I recoup year by year is a combination of the saving on my energy bill and the surplus energy I sell back to the national grid.

If I recoup 5% of what I originally paid for installation, i, in the first year, that means that 5% of the installation cost was equal to the saving on energy bills in the first year, x, and the number of kilowatt hours I gave back to the national grid, k, multiplied by 0.1 (to get an answer in pounds).

In other words $0.05i = x + 0.1k$

I know I sold back 5000 kWh, so I got $0.1 \times 5000 = £500$ for the energy I sold back to the grid, so $0.05i = x + 500$

In the second year, I recouped an additional $11.25 - 5 = 6.25\%$ of the installation costs. My energy bills in the second year would have been the same as my energy bills last year. I sold 7500 kWh of energy to the grid, so I received £750. So, $0.0625i = x + 750$

Therefore, solving simultaneous equations:

$0.0625i - 0.05i = 0.0125i = 750 - 500 + x - x = 250$

$250/0.0125 = £20,000$

30. Answer = A

To calculate the distance, we can work out the area under the graph.

Car V travels at a constant speed for the entire 60 seconds – this is equivalent to a straight line on the graph. Therefore, Car V travels $5 \times 60 = 300$ m.

For Car S you need to calculate the distance travelled during the first 10 seconds, then the remaining 50 seconds. For the first 10 seconds Car S travelled: $20 \times 10 \times 0.5 = 100$ m. For the remaining 50 seconds car S travelled: $20 \times 50 = 1000$ m. The total distance travelled by Car S in 60 seconds is $1000 + 100$ m $= 1100$ m.

The difference is: $1100 - 300 = 800$, so Car S travelled 800 m further than Car V.

31. Answer = D

The passage states that the ruling is 'fundamentally unfair because careful female drivers are now effectively subsidising their young and reckless male counterparts'. Yet, if 'D' were true, this would not be correct, as the fact that male drivers are more likely to suffer a crash that leads to serious injury or death would no longer be particularly relevant to arguments about premiums.

A is incorrect because it is not relevant to the argument presented.

B is incorrect because the argument does not state that drivers exclusively drive in one way.

C is incorrect because, while it suggests that prior to the ruling male drivers were subsidising women drivers, it does not weaken the argument that female drivers are being penalised now.

E is incorrect because the argument is concerned with young male drivers being subsidised; this point relates only to those over 35.

32. Answer = C

To start, calculate the number of doctors and nurses currently employed:

- Nurses = 480 × 55% = 264
- Doctors = 480 × 20% = 96

Then calculate the number of doctors and nurses after the additional 100 staff are employed:

- Nurses = (480 + 100) × 55% = 319
- Doctors = (480 + 100) × 20% = 116

The final step is to add the number of new doctors and nurses = (319 – 264) + (116 – 96) = 55 + 20 = 75.

33. Answer = E

A: Incorrect as the initial three digits are different (these represent the clinic code).

B: Incorrect as the 4/5 digits represent the day of the month which can therefore not be larger than 31

C: Incorrect as the 6/7 digits represent the month which can therefore not be larger than 12

D: Incorrect as the security code should be 10 (125 – 22 = 103 / 10 = 10.3 = 10)

E: Correct

34. Answer = C

You know that each candle burns for 20 minutes, so by lighting one candle you can measure 20 minutes (as well as 40 and 60 minutes as you have three candles).

If you were to light a candle from both ends simultaneously, it would burn in 10 minutes. You can therefore measure 10, 20 and 30 minutes using this technique, or by combining with lighting some from one end measure 10, 20, 30, 40, 50 or 60 minutes.

It is also possible to measure 15 minutes. Light two candles: one from one end and the other from both ends. Once the candle lit from both ends has burnt out (10 minutes) then light the second end of the first candle – which will now finish burning in 5 minutes. This will make 15 minutes in total.

Note that as you only have three candles the maximum time period you can measure is 60 minutes.

35.   Answer = A

The passage states that 'in the Western world the idea of polygamy is seen as ... morally wrong'. But it goes on to say that, in 'other parts of the world', polygamy is 'viewed as a positive, rather than a negative, domestic dynamic'. By doing this, the passage demonstrates the difficulty of applying moral judgement on a global scale.

B is incorrect because the passage does not evaluate the limitations of marriage in the Western world.

C is incorrect because the passage does not attempt to make an argument either way; it merely highlights two conflicting stances.

D is incorrect because the passage is balanced and does not attack or defend a position. Nor is polygamy shown to be 'universally' seen one way or the other.

E is incorrect as the passage does not offer any evaluations or conclusions. It only draws attention to perceptions.

Section 2

Answer Key:

Question	Answer
1	C
2	G
3	C
4	A
5	B
6	B
7	D
8	E
9	A
10	D
11	C
12	D
13	B
14	A
15	A
16	C
17	D
18	A
19	E
20	C
21	B
22	B
23	D
24	C
25	D
26	D
27	E

Score Conversion:

Total Score	Suggested BMAT Score
0	1.0
1	1.0
2	1.0
3	1.5
4	2.1
5	2.6
6	3.1
7	3.6
8	4.0
9	4.4
10	4.7
11	4.9
12	5.1
13	5.3
14	5.6
15	5.9
16	6.2
17	6.5
18	6.8
19	7.1
20	7.5
21	8.0
22	8.5
23	9.0
24	9.0
25	9.0
26	9.0
27	9.0

1. Answer = C

If individual C is heterozygous and *expresses* the illness, the disease must be dominant. This means, if his daughters do *not* express the illness, they must both be homozygous recessive.

If individual B is heterozygous and has a child with a homozygous recessive partner, the chance that the child will have the disease is 50%.

If individual C is homozygous, and if his daughters do *not* express the disease, he must be homozygous recessive. Moreover, if his daughters do not express the disease, they must be heterozygous. Individual B must also be homozygous recessive to express the illness. The chance of a homozygous recessive individual having a child that expresses the trait with a heterozygous individual is also 50%.

2. Answer = G

None of the three statements is correct.

A) Incorrect: polymerisation occurs between alkene monomers. Alkenes discolour bromine water, not hydrogen bromide – which is colourless anyway.

B) Incorrect: monomers must be *un*saturated hydrocarbons.

C) Incorrect: although the first two molecules could be monomers, $C_2H_4Cl_2$ could not be a monomer because it would be completely saturated (i.e. no double bond between the carbons).

3. Answer = C

If 3.6 dm³ of carbon monoxide is reacted, there must be 3.6/24 = 0.15 moles of carbon monoxide being reacted. This means that we will get 2/3 × 0.15 = 0.1 moles of Fe. Therefore, the total mass of Fe that we will end up with is 0.1 × 56 = 5.6 g.

4. Answer = A

Only answer option A is correct:

A) Correct: one mole of sodium-22 will have a mass of 22/1 = 22 g. Five years is equal to two half-lives, so the mass of sodium-22 in the sample will halve then halve again: 22 × 0.5 × 0.5 = 5.5 g.

B) Incorrect: In *positron* beta-decay, a proton changes into a neutron. Hence the new atomic number will be 10 and the atomic mass will remain unchanged at 22. The difference is therefore 12.

C) Incorrect: as the new atomic number is 10, the newly formed element will also have 10 electrons. This gives it the same electronic configuration as neon, a noble gas that is inert.

5. Answer = B

$$P = 1 - \sqrt{\frac{n^2 + a}{n + a}}$$

$$\sqrt{\frac{n^2 + a}{n + a}} = 1 - P$$

$$\frac{n^2 + a}{n + a} = (1 - P)^2$$

$n^2 + a = (1 - P)^2(n + a)$

$n^2 + a = n(1 - P)^2 + a(1 - P)^2$

$a - a(1 - P)^2 = n(1 - P)^2 - n^2$

$a(1 - (1 - P)^2) = n(1 - P)^2 - n^2$

$a = \dfrac{n(1-P)^2 - n^2}{1-(1-P)^2}$

6. Answer = B

Remember that $1\,L = 1\,dm^3 = 1000\,cm^3$.

Eventually, the mass of the drug will be dissolved in a volume of fluid equal to the volume of the blood and the volume of the fluid in the drip bag: $5 + 0.5 = 5.5\,L = 5.5\,dm^3$.

The concentration of the drug in the body is given by *moles* $\div 5.5 = 0.1$ mmoldm³.

- $1\,moldm^{-3} = 1000\,mmoldm^{-3}$
- So $1\,mmoldm^{-3} = 0.001\,moldm^{-3}$
- $0.1\,mmoldm^{-3} = 0.0001\,moldm^{-3}$
- Therefore, *moles* $= 0.0001 \times 5.5 = 0.00055$

The moles of the drug required is given by *mass* $\div 300 = 0.00055$. Therefore, the mass of the drug required is $0.00055 \times 300 = 0.165$ g.

7. Answer = D

A. Incorrect: ligase *sticks together* genetic material.

B. Incorrect: human insulin produced by GM bacteria is used to treat diabetics. Normal bacteria don't produce insulin!

C. Incorrect: the insulin *gene* is inserted into bacterial plasmids. Insulin as a word by itself refers to the *protein*.

D. Correct: normally, a human cell contains two copies of every gene (one on each chromosome copy). During mitosis, the amount of genetic material in the cell doubles. Hence there is a point in the cell cycle where it contains four copies of every gene.

E. Incorrect: ligase is an enzyme; increasing the temperature of ligase indefinitely will eventually cause it to denature.

8. Answer = E

When both objects were held at 5 m above the ground, they both had potential energy of $5 \times 10 \times m = 50m$ joules (where m is the identical mass of each object).

At time t, object A has potential energy of $4 \times 10 \times m = 40m$ joules (PE = mgh). As it has fallen in a vacuum, all of its potential energy *must* have been converted into kinetic energy. Therefore it has $50 - 40 = 10m$ joules of kinetic energy. Since kinetic energy is equal to ½ mv^2, its velocity must equal:

- $10m = \frac{1}{2} mv^2$
- $20 = v^2$
- $v = \sqrt{20} = 2\sqrt{5}$ ms^{-1}
- Similarly, at time t object B has $30m$ joules of potential energy, $20m$ joules of kinetic energy, and a velocity of $\sqrt{40} = 2\sqrt{10}$ ms^{-1}

A. Incorrect: $2\sqrt{10}$ ms^{-1} > $2\sqrt{5}$ ms^{-1}, so B is moving faster.

B. Incorrect: object B has less potential energy than object A.

C. Incorrect: the objects are falling in a vacuum, so no energy will be lost as heat due to drag.

D. Incorrect: the kinetic energy of each object will simply be equal to the lost potential energy.

E. Correct: If the velocity of object B is $2\sqrt{10}$ ms^{-1} and the velocity of A is $2\sqrt{5}$ ms^{-1} then object B is moving at a velocity that is greater than object A's velocity by a factor of $2\sqrt{10} \div 2\sqrt{5} = \sqrt{10}/\sqrt{5} = \sqrt{2}$ times faster.

9. Answer = A

Set up a series of simultaneous equations and solve:

- For moles of H: $2a + b = 2 + 2d$
- For moles of S: $a = 1$
- For moles of O: $4a = d$
- For moles of I: $b = 2c$

So $2 + b = 2 + 2d$

$b = 2d = 2c$

$d = 4$

$c = 4$

$b = 8$

10. Answer = D

Assessing each option in turn:

1. Correct – when $2x^2 + 3 = x + 3$, $0 = x(1 - 2x)$. Hence, $x = 0$ when the two lines cross and the corresponding coordinate is $(0,3)$.

2. Correct – $f(x - 1) = 2(x - 1)^2 + 3 = 2(x^2 - 2x + 1) + 3 = 2x^2 - 4x + 5$.

3. Incorrect – $f(x - 1) = 2x^2 - 4x + 5$, but it represents a translation of 1 along the x-axis, not $- 1$.

11. Answer = C

Neuronal signals travel along neurons – they are elicited at the nerve cell dendrites and then travel along the length of the axon. In a reflex arc, the correct order in which the signal moves is:

Receptor tissue → sensory neuron → interneuron → motor neuron → effector tissue

12. Answer = D

The container should be made from *wood*, because wood is a better thermal insulator than metal.

Its interior and exterior should be shiny, because shiny surfaces are poor absorbers and emitters of heat.

We will not be able to absorb heat from the surroundings, because the tea will be hotter than the surroundings. Hence we do not need a matt exterior to absorb ambient surrounding heat. Instead, we want to slow down heat *loss*.

13. Answer = B

From the description, we know the type of organic substance we are dealing with is a carboxylic acid. The combined masses in the empirical formula come to $(12 \times 2) + 16 + (4 \times 1)$ = 44. Therefore, the molecule has a formula of $C_4O_2H_8$. As it has four carbons, it must be butanoic acid.

14. Answer = A

A. Incorrect: If a cell is placed into distilled water, calcium ions will move out of it *down* their concentration gradient.

B. Correct: if a cell is placed in 2 mmolL^{-1} calcium ion solution, protein X has to move ions against a larger concentration gradient, so its energy consumption will increase.

C. Correct: the extracellular solution is more dilute than the cytoplasm, so water will move inwards by diffusion.

D. Correct: as above.

E. Correct: 1 mmolL^{-1} = 1000 μmolL^{-1}. Therefore 1000 ÷ 0.1 = 10,000.

15. Answer = A

There are several ways I could pick out two reds and a blue:

1. I could pick out a red first, then a blue, then another red (then I would have to stop).

2. I could pick out a red first, then another red, then a blue, then a green.

The probability of situation 1 happening is $1/3 \times 3/8 \times 2/7 = 1/28$

The probability of situation 2 happening is $1/3 \times 2/8 \times 3/7 \times 3/6 = 1/56$

So the overall probability of getting two red balls and a single blue ball is $1/28 + 1/56 = 3/56$

16. Answer = C

A. Correct: as the object moves towards the speaker, it will encounter sound waves in quicker succession than if it was stationary. In other words, for the object the time period of the waves will seem shorter. As time period is inversely proportional to frequency, it will encounter higher-frequency sound waves.

B. Correct: $330/1650 = 0.2$ m; $3 \times 10^8/3 \times 10^{10} = 0.01$ m. Remember, 300,000 km/s $= 3 \times 10^8$ m/s and that 1 GHz $= 1 \times 10^9$ Hz.

C. Incorrect: Sound waves *are* longitudinal. However, by definition, if a wave travels through a medium the particles in that medium do *not* undergo a *net* displacement due to the wave. Hence the air particles in this scenario would in fact oscillate around a fixed position in a movement that is parallel to the direction of travel of the wave.

D. Correct: ultrasound imaging of foetuses, for instance.

E. Correct: due to the Doppler effect, the sound waves that reach the person will have spread out and will be perceived at a lower frequency than the frequency at which they are emitted by the loudspeaker. So the person will perceive a lower tone than is produced by the loudspeaker, and the loudspeaker will be producing a tone that is higher than that perceived by the person.

17. Answer = D

A. Incorrect: structure 1 is the salivary glands. These produce saliva containing *amylase* but not *protease* (which would digest the mouth!).

B. Incorrect: stomach acid forms part of the *innate* immune system.

C. Incorrect: structure 2 shows the oesophagus, but it is the *trachea* that is maintained by C-shaped rings of cartilage.

D. Correct: structure 6 indicates the jejunum.

E. Incorrect: structure 11, the gall bladder, receives bile synthesised by the liver, structure 12, and secretes it into the small intestine.

18. Answer = A

We are looking at a sequence; it is clear that the differences between the terms are not constant (they are 2, 5, 8 and 11). However, the differences between the differences are all 3. Hence the size of the area on a particular day can be described as part of a quadratic sequence.

As the difference between the differences is 3, the expression for the sequence must contain $1.5n^2$.

The differences between the terms in the sequence and the corresponding $1.5n^2$ parts is

$5 - 1.5(1^2) = 3.5$

$7 - 1.5(2^2) = 1$

$12 - 1.5(3^2) = -1.5$

$20 - 1.5(4^2) = -4$

$31 - 1.5(5^2) = -6.5$

Hence the expression for the nth term contains the arithmetic sequence $-2.5n + 6$.

So overall, the expression is $1.5n^2 - 2.5n + 6$.

Therefore, on day 30, the patch will have an area of $1.5(30^2) - 2.5 \times 30 + 6 = 1281$ mm^2.

19. Answer = E

Both statements B and C are correct:

A) Incorrect: resistors R2 and R3 are arranged in series with each other, but in parallel to resistor R1. Therefore, the total resistance of the resistors in the 'parallel' part of the circuit can be found out from $1/R_{para} = 1/R1 + 1/(R2 + R3)$. So R_{para} is $(R1 + R2 + R3) \div R1(R2 + R3)$.

Resistors R1, R2 and R3 are arranged in series to resistor R4, so the total resistance of the circuit is $(R_{para} + R4)$.

The current shown by A1 and A2 *will* be equal, but it will be equal to $V \div (R_{para} + R4) =$ $V \div ((R1 + R2 + R3)/R1(R2 + R3)) = VR1(R2 + R3) \div (R1 + R2 + R3)$.

B) Correct: we are told in the question that *fixed* resistors are used in the circuit. Therefore, the resistance will remain constant regardless of the voltage across the resistor.

C) Correct: resistance multiplied by current will give us the voltage across the component. A definition of voltage is the amount of work that is performed on each unit of charge to move it through a component. A volt can also be written as a joule per coulomb.

20. Answer = C

Only answer option, C, is correct:

A) Incorrect: the ionic half-equation should be $Cu^{2+} + 2e^- \rightarrow Cu$

B) Incorrect: if a copper anode is placed in copper (II) sulfate solution and a voltage is applied, the anode will be positively charged and *lose* Cu^{2+} ions into the solution. Gradually, it will decrease in size.

C) Correct: the reaction in the equation is a displacement reaction showing that zinc is more reactive than copper. If carbon is more reactive than zinc, carbon will therefore be more reactive than copper.

21. Answer = B

Only answer option, B, is correct:

A) Incorrect: we can tell from the question that the patient is female. Therefore it cannot be a Y-linked disorder!

B) Correct: during anaerobic exercise, glucose is converted to lactate. Lactate is then converted into CO_2 by reacting it with oxygen. If the patient is less able to transport oxygen, this second process will be impaired.

C) Incorrect: an increase in lactate, or lactic acid, following a period of anaerobic exercise will lead to blood having a *lower* pH. So as lactate will persist in the patient's blood for longer than in a healthy individual, her pH will remain *lowered* for longer.

22. Answer = B

It is pushed at a constant speed across a horizontal surface, so the driving force acting upon it must be equal to the friction acting upon it. Hence the driving force is also 40 kN.

Work = force × distance, so 1,000,000 = 40,000 × distance (m)

Distance = 1,000,000/40,000 = 25 m

Note that the weight of the block is not needed to answer the question.

23. Answer = D

If a catalyst is used, the reaction will have a faster rate. However, if the temperature is raised, the endothermic direction of the reaction will be favoured and *less* ammonia will be produced at equilibrium. Therefore we are looking for the graph with a steeper initial gradient, but a smaller plateau, than the one in the question. Only Graph D fulfils these criteria.

24. Answer = C

Only answer option, C, is correct:

A) Incorrect: note that the scores of the *three highest-scoring students* were removed. This means that the average of these students' scores, a, *must* be greater than the average score of the rest of the candidates.

B) Incorrect: the median score *might* change; therefore this statement cannot *definitely* be true. If it helps, create a thought experiment to see if you can identify when the median score would change. For instance, if the scores happened to be

1, 1, 2, 3, 3, 5, 7, 8, 9

then the median is initially 3. However, if the top 3 marks are removed then the median changes to 2.5.

C) Correct: the total score, including the scores of the cheaters, is given by $T(x + y)$. The cheaters scored an average of a, so in total they got a combined score of $3a$. So the *new* total score for the test once the cheaters' marks are removed is $T(x + y) - 3a$. To work out the new average, we just have to divide that by the number of non-cheating students, $x + y - 3$.

25. Answer = D

A. Three free neutrons are released as a result of the nuclear fission of uranium-235.

B. Uranium-236 is produced momentarily in the nuclear fission chain reaction of uranium-235 when the nucleus of a uranium-235 absorbs one of the free neutrons that was produced by a previous fission event.

C. Both nuclear fusion and fission release heat energy (usually in large quantities).

D. Deuterium is a hydrogen isotope of mass 2 that can be fused with a hydrogen-1 isotope to produce helium-3. It will not be produced as a result of the fusion of hydrogen, because the resulting atom will have too many protons in its nucleus.

E. Krypton-90 is a possible by-product of the fission of uranium-235. An unstable uranium-236 nucleus may split to form krypton-90 and barium-143.

F.   Helium-3 is the product of a fusion between deuterium and hydrogen-1.

26.   Answer = D

A.   Incorrect: we can see that amino acids are produced in nutrient mixtures B and C after treatment with Preparation 3, so Preparation 3 must contain enzymes. Preparation 2 is in fact the saline solution since it elicits no change.

B.   Incorrect: we know that nutrient mixture A contains glucose from the start. However, because amylase breaks down starch into glucose, we cannot know for sure if mixture A contains starch with this method (glucose produced from starch is non-distinguishable from pre-existing glucose in this case).

C.   Incorrect: we know that B contains starch, because after treatment with preparation A glucose was present in the mixture when it hadn't been previously. We also know it contains protein, because amino acids were produced for the first time after the addition of preparation 3. However, we cannot know for sure if mixture B contained fat too, because glycerol was present in B from the start, and this would have hidden the presence of glycerol produced by the breakdown of fat.

D.   Correct: preparation 1 elicits the production of glycerol from C, so C must contain fat (and 1 must contain lipase). Preparation 3 elicits the production of amino acids, so C must contain protein as well (and 3 must contain protease).

E.   Incorrect: if this was true, we would expect to find amino acids in all three mixtures (A, B and C) after treatment; however, none is present in mixture A so this cannot be the case.

27.   Answer = E

A.   Correct: an object with circular motion will have a constantly changing velocity, because it is changing direction constantly (in which case it will be accelerating). However, it may still be moving at a constant speed.

B.   Correct: if the train is moving on straight rails its direction cannot change. Therefore a change in velocity can only come from a change in speed.

C.   Correct: if an object is falling at terminal velocity, the vertical forces acting upon it must be balanced. However, horizontal forces may still be unbalanced. (Imagine a skydiver with an open parachute, falling at terminal velocity. A breeze may still push her horizontally, even though she maintains a falling terminal velocity.)

D.   Correct: work done is equal to the force applied to an object multiplied by the distance that is moved in the direction of that force. The force will be proportional to the mass of the object, since $F = ma$. Hence:

$W = F \times d = m \times a \times d$, so work done will be proportional to the mass of the object.

E.   Incorrect: an object of mass 10 g will have a weight of $0.01 \times 10 = 0.1$ N acting upon it. This is not balanced with the drag of 100 N, so the object will decelerate.

Section 3

1. 'The medical profession, after all, deals partly with guess work; we do not deal in absolutes.' Paul Beeson, MD

Explain what this statement means. Argue that there are times when the medical profession does deal with absolutes. To what extent do you agree that the medical profession deals partly with guesswork?

Notes

Explain it

Key terms:

Partly – To an extent

Deals in – Is predicated upon

Guess work – Things we do not know for certain

Absolutes – Things that are beyond dispute

Therefore:

Paul Beeson is saying that the medical profession is, to an extent, predicated upon things we do not know for certain. It is not based solely on things that are beyond dispute. (32 words)

Argue objectively

Arguments to the contrary, i.e. where the medical profession DOES deal with absolutes:

- Raised blood pressure readings following 24-hour monitoring.
- You either have a condition, or you do not.
- Histological diagnosis of tumour cells for bowel cancer.

Express an opinion

Arguments for the medical profession dealing partly with guesswork.

- Appendicitis cannot be diagnosed with 100% accuracy prior to operation.
- Psychiatric conditions.

Conclusion

In theory, there are no absolutes.

Much of medicine is based on very informed guesswork, founded upon experience.

Sample answer

Paul Beeson is saying that the medical profession is, to an extent, predicated upon things we do not know for certain. It is not based solely on things that are beyond dispute.

However, there are times when a doctor does need to deal in absolutes. For instance, when checking whether someone has raised blood pressure, their readings are monitored for 24 hours. If the readings are above an absolute numerical level, they are considered to have high blood pressure. While where the cut-off is set can be disputed, the number cannot.

The clearest example of 'absolutes' in medicine arises when someone either has a condition, or they do not. In the histological diagnosis of tumour cells for bowel cancer, a result will be returned that says that the patient either does, or does not, have bowel cancer.

In the most extreme instance, someone is either alive or dead.

However, Paul Beeson does have a valid point when he suggests that part of medicine is based on guesswork.

If there is a strong suspicion of appendicitis, a patient will often undergo the operation to remove their appendix. This is because there is no categorical way to exclude the possibility of appendicitis. The operation is therefore based on the suspicions – or best guess – of the doctor.

There are some medical fields that are predicated more on guesswork than others. Psychiatry is a good example of this. Since there often no visible symptoms of psychiatric disorders, they can be extremely difficult to diagnose with certainty. Therefore, psychiatrists must use their insights to provide an informed opinion – or best guess.

In theory, there are no absolutes. There is always a chance of human error – whether it is in diagnosing diseases of the body, the mind, or even in pronouncing someone dead. To that extent, doctors are always partaking in 'guesswork'.

The responsibility of a good doctor is to make his or her guesses as informed as possible, based on years of training and experience.

2. 'A man who cannot work without his hypodermic needle is a poor doctor. The amount of narcotic you use is inversely proportional to your skill.' Martin H. Fischer

Explain the argument behind this statement. Argue to the contrary, that the use of narcotics does not suggest a lack of medical skill. To what extent do you agree that being able to work without a hypodermic needle is the sign of a skilful doctor?

Notes

Explain it

Key terms:

'A man' – in this context, a doctor

'Cannot' – unable

'Hypodermic needle' – means of administering drugs

'Narcotic' – drugs/medications

'Inversely proportional to your skill' – the more you do it, the less skill you have

Therefore:

Martin Fischer is suggesting that a doctor unable to work without administering drugs is bad at their job, and that those who administer large amounts of drugs have less skill than those who administer less. (35 words)

Argue objectively

Arguments to the contrary, i.e. that the use of narcotics does not represent a lack of skill:

- Narcotics are a very important part of medicine.
- Some fields, like anaesthesia, rely more heavily on narcotics than others.
- Administering of narcotics is a very precise skill, e.g. controlling blood pressure.

Express an opinion

Arguments for being able to work without a hypodermic needle being the mark of a good doctor:

- Some doctors might be over-reliant on narcotics at the expense of other skills.
- Overuse of drugs has negative consequences, e.g. resistance.

Conclusion

Narcotics are necessary but should be used sensibly.

Good doctors know when and how to administer.

Sample answer

Martin Fischer is suggesting that a doctor unable to work without administering drugs is bad at their job, and that those who administer large amounts of drugs have less skill than those who administer less.

However, there are many cases where the administering of large amounts of narcotics to various patients does not represent a lack of skill.

Narcotics are a very important part of modern medicine. They can be used to control and cure ailments that otherwise would progress to the detriment of the patient. For example, drugs are often used to control blood pressure. This has many benefits, such as reducing the chances of suffering a stroke.

There are also some medical fields that rely more heavily on the administering of narcotics than others. For example, the job of the anaesthetist is to administer drugs so that the patient remains unconscious during serious operations. In this case, the ability to do this well is the mark of a good doctor – not of a bad one.

In general medicine, the administering of narcotics is extremely important. Being able to give the right doses of the right drugs in the right situation is a precise art.

Nonetheless, Fischer does raise an important point. Many doctors might be considered to rely too heavily upon the administering of narcotics. This might be to the detriment of other skills that a good doctor should have, such as providing a precise diagnosis.

In some cases, using drugs where they are unnecessary might have undesirable consequences. For instance, if antibiotics are given too readily when they are not needed, harmful bacteria can develop resistance to them.

In conclusion, narcotics are a necessary and important part of modern medicine. However, they should be used sensibly. The skill of a good doctor comes in knowing when to use narcotics, and when not to, in order to benefit the patient.

Index

and nuclear fusion, 105, 178, 202

    oxidation number, 71

hydrogenation, 67, 81

hydrogen bonding, 82

hydrogen halides, 82

hydrogen ions, 75, 79

hydroxide ions, 75, 79

hypotenuse, 119

I

immiscible liquids, 75

immune system, 53, 59, 173, 200

index laws, 106–7

inequalities, 112

infrared radiation, 98, 101, 173

insulation, 85, 97, 171, 199

insulin, 47, 57, 170, 197

interior angles, 117–18, 123

interquartile range, 129

iodide ions, 68

ion exchange membrane, 75–6

ionic bonding, 63

ionic equations, 68, 70–1, 201

ionic lattice structures, 64

ions, 62–4

    charge on common, 69

iron, 65–7, 69, 169

isotopes, 63, 105, 169

IUPAC (International Union of Pure and Applied Chemistry), 80

K

key terms, 141–2, 148, 204, 206

kidneys, *see* renal system

kinetic energy, 77, 95–8, 170, 197–8

L

lactate, 51, 175, 201

language, objective and subjective, 144–5, 147

LCM (lowest common multiple), 106

LH (luteinising hormone), 58

ligase, 47, 170, 197

light

    as energy, 96

    speed of, 100

    visible, 101–2

linear equations, 114

line graphs, 26, 114, 125

line of best fit, 128

liquids, 39, 68–9, 74–6, 96–8

lithium, 66–7

logical reasoning, 18, 20–3, 25

longitudinal waves, 98, 100

loop of Henle, 56

lower quartile, 126–7, 129

M

magnesium, 65–6, 71, 103

magnitude, orders of, 28

mass, use of term, 94

mathematical reasoning, 18

matter, phases of, 96–7

mean, 128, 163, 191

median, 126–9, 177, 202

The Medic Portal, xii, 34

meiosis, 39–41, 45

menstrual cycle, 57

metal extraction, 65

metallic bonding, 63

metals

    and acids, 80

    alkali, 66–8

    and covalent structures, 64

    and displacement reactions, 66

    oxidation numbers of, 70

    in periodic table, 65

    transition, 67, 69

microvilli, 55

microwaves, 101

miscible liquids, 74

mitosis, 39, 41, 197

mode, 129